NURSING HISTORY:
The State of the Art

Edited by
Christopher Maggs

CROOM HELM
London • Sydney • Wolfeboro, New Hampshire

© 1987 Christopher J. Maggs.
Chapter 7 © 1985 Aspen Publications, Inc.
Croom Helm Ltd, Provident House, Burrell Row,
Beckenham, Kent BR3 1AT
Croom Helm, 44–50 Waterloo Road, North Ryde,
2113, NSW, Australia

British Library Cataloguing in Publication Data

Nursing history : the state of the art.
1. Nursing — History
I. Maggs, Christopher J.
610.73'09   RT31

ISBN 0-7099-4637-6

Croom Helm, 27 South Main Street,
Wolfeboro, New Hampshire 03894–2069, USA

Library of Congress Cataloging-in-Publication Data

Nursing history.

Includes index.
1. Nursing — History. I. Maggs, Christopher J.
(DNLM: 1. History of nursing. WY 11 N974)
RT31.N874 1987   610.73'09   86-32802
ISBN 0-7099-4637-6 (pbk.)

Phototypeset by Sunrise Setting, Torquay, Devon
Printed and bound in Great Britain by Mackays of Chatham Ltd, Kent

Contents

List of Contributors
Acknowledgements

List of Contributors

Christopher Maggs is currently the Royal National Pension Fund for Nurses's Visiting Fellow at the Wellcome Unit for the History of Medicine, Oxford. He is writing the centennial history of the Fund; in addition, he is the author of a modular component on nursing history for the Open Tech. and Editor of *History of Nursing Bulletin*. The author of many articles on the history of nursing, his first book, *Origins of General Nursing* was published in 1983 (reprinted 1985) by Croom Helm.

Josephine Castle, Lecturer in History, Wollongong University, NSW, is the author of several articles on Australian and women's history. Her most recent publication is 'Women Workers at Courtaulds and GEC, 1920–1939' in T. Mason and B. Lancaster (eds), *Life and Labour in Twentieth-Century Coventry*.

Monica E. Baly is the well-known nursing historian and Fellow of the Royal College of Nursing. She is currently working on a study of the history of the Queen's Nursing Institute nurses.

Sidney D. Krampitz is Professor, Dept of Psychiatry-Mental Health Nursing and Assistant Dean and Director of Graduate Programmes at the University of Kansas School of Nursing, College of Health Sciences, Kansas City, Kansas. She is the author of several articles on the history of nursing and power relationships in nursing.

Alice Friedman, now retired, is Professor Emeritus at the University of Massachusetts, Amherst, USA. Active in nursing history and archive preservation, she is on the editorial board of the *Journal of Nursing History*.

Ruth Hawker, Senior Tutor at the Royal Devon and Exeter Hospital, has published several articles on patients and their relatives. She is an adviser to the Florence Nightingale Museum at St Thomas's Hospital, London.

Olga Maranjian Church is Assistant Professor at the University of Illinois College of Nursing. She is active in nursing history affairs and is the author of several articles on nursing and nursing politics.

Laura Linebach, RN, BSN, is both a nurse and an air stewardess teacher for TWA. She is also a freelance writer and Chairperson of the Nursing Heritage Foundation, Kansas City, Kansas. Her most recent publication is *From Lily to Lanie: The History of the VNA of Greater Kansas City*.

Cynthia Q. Woods is a doctoral student at the University of Kansas School of Nursing, Kansas City, Kansas.

Acknowledgements

The editor and publishers wish to thank the following for permission to reprint:

The Editors, *History of Nursing Bulletin*, Royal College of Nursing, London for permission to reprint Sidney D. Krampitz, 'The Yale Experiment: Innovation in Nursing Education', *History of Nursing Bulletin*, no. 8 (Autumn 1985).

Aspen Publishers, 1600 Research Boulevard, Rockville, MD, 20850, USA, for permission to reprint Olga Maranjian Church, 'The Emergence of Training Programmes for Asylum Nursing at the turn of the Century' from *Advances in Nursing Science* (Nursing History Edition), vol. 7, no.2 (January 1985).

1

Nursing History: Contemporary Practice and Contemporary Concerns

Christopher Maggs

This present collection of articles may be regarded in some ways as a sequel to the innovative volume edited by Celia Davies (1981), *Rewriting Nursing History*. It takes up some of the challenges and questions posed in that work and seeks to show whether the rewriting of nursing history has continued as Davies and her fellow contributors hoped it would. It is also an answer to an observation made some time later by Davies: asked if the time was right for a sequel, she wondered whether there was sufficient new nursing history being written to justify another volume. The collection of articles assembled here demonstrates that her worries were groundless. Two of the contributions have been published elsewhere but they and the other original pieces now have this opportunity of reaching a wider audience.

We are witnessing an exciting era in nursing and nursing history, and the tide of new writings looks set to become a flood. The variety of topics which this volume covers shows that radical approaches to conventional themes run alongside the discovery of new paths for nursing history. Several of the contributors reassess received conventions, pointing out the historiographical problems in the writing of nursing history; others broaden the concerns of nursing history by looking at new and hitherto unexplored questions. Taken together, they illustrate the state of the art in nursing history and confirm Celia Davies's belief, expressed in 1981, that there is a new commitment among historians of nursing to develop 'diverse approaches' and question ' an orthodox history of nursing'.[1]

THE 'PROBLEM' OF NURSING HISTORY OR THE HISTORY OF NURSING

It comes as something of a shock to realise that the question — is there something which can be called nursing history? — has not really been asked.[2] There appears to be an assumption among those taking part that what they are producing *is* nursing history, or that they are working in a field called 'nursing history'. It may, of course, be that the question is irrelevant. What is important is that nursing is critically examined in all its aspects, including the historical. On the other hand, some writers use the phrase — the history of nursing — and we are left wondering if that is the same as or in some significant way different from nursing history. Should we use capital letters when writing such titles?

Michael Carpenter, an exception to this generalisation, has taken a firm line on this point. He argues that the idea 'of a separate nursing history is itself ideologically loaded . . . An insular nursing history implicitly seeks to stake out the social distance between nurses, other kinds of health workers and the working class in general.'[3] Since he rejects the 'reification' of nursing and general nursing specifically, he also rejects 'the idea of a separate history of nursing, simply regarding it as one chapter in the history of labour.'[4] Carpenter's work on asylum nurses certainly put nurses back into nursing history — by looking at their origins; motivation; class characteristics and allegiances; unionisation and industrial militancy — but is his argument for it to be *simply* a chapter in the history of labour sufficient?

Histories of nursing generally began to appear from the mid-nineteenth century onwards, many being published in the 1880s and 1890s. These early works were prompted by the nursing reform movements and were either accounts of the introduction of reforms, biographical studies of reformers, or glorifications of a past era of nursing which, it was argued, needed to be rediscovered to lift nursing out of the dark ages. In a real sense, they were celebratory histories, written by those who were actively engaged in the reform movements or who were supportive of them.[5] As Davies points out, nursing history tends to 'focus upon individuals, leaders in the field, exceptional people who struggle against the odds and win. And it is evaluative, indeed largely congratulatory, in so far as it sees the history of nursing as an advance, as progress out of the dark ages to the present, modern times.'[6]

A dichotomy exists in this broad consensus: Katherine Williams has identified the distinction between histories of nursing written by nurses or nurse-orientated writers and those by doctors and others who shared their world views.[7] On the one hand, 'In the nursing view, the old methods have been supplanted by a new system, which is regarded as that upon which occupational identity should be properly based.' On the other, 'The medical view agrees that there is a new system, but is unsatisfied with its content and disturbed by the attempt to create from it a unified occupational identity.'[8] The first group were, in the main, women writers; the second, men. Both accounts, however, agree that nursing has been reformed and is developing towards the modern. The bases for this split are to be found in gender and class relationships as much as in pragmatic acknowledgement of nursing's relative position to medicine in the nineteenth century. They also reflect an underlying power struggle within health care. Doctors urgently needed more nurses to meet the demands they were creating as medicine expanded and preferred to develop training programmes which would produce competent nurses as quickly as possible. Nurse leaders wanted to educate nurses, not just to train them; they favoured a more systematic and structured approach to nurse education.

Not all of these histories are 'insular', however. Even where their subject is treated without reference to a larger canvas of social experience, or without the benefits of comparative data and analyses, they are informed by specific concerns which are themselves the product of identifiable ideologies. For example, biographical studies of nursing leaders, including Florence Nightingale, serve to document the 'rise' of nursing and at the same time to illuminate contemporary debates about such issues as women's social position; women's work and the division of labour; the family; and power relationships. That most authors neglect or were unable to indicate the theoretical arguments, should not lead us to suppose that they were unaware of or not involved in them. What we do have to acknowledge, if we look at who actually wrote those accounts, was the close involvement by many 'historians' in the political and occupational struggles within and surrounding nursing. Their histories were written as political statements and not just as rather self-congratulatory pieces of rhetoric.

That does not mean, however, that those histories represent

'the history' of nursing. What it does mean is that part of each generation of nurse historians is seeking to discuss nursing with specific and differing objectives in mind. We are no longer concerned with the issue of regulation and state registration in Britain. Nursing historians, then, have no need to write their histories in order to sustain a campaign for state registration for nurses. They may well want to write about the consequences of regulation on the occupation — loss of autonomy; exclusion of groups of health workers; the emphasis on professional rather than union organisations, and so on. But purposes and ends change.

But it is not this aspect of nursing history which really worries writers like Carpenter. He would accept that some, perhaps all, historical accounts are written with both overt and covert biases and purposes. What seems to be of most concern is the real possibility that such historical accounts will assume the status of a model for nurses themselves. And it is the fascination for and concentration on general nursing and general hospitals by nursing historians which is most often criticised. As Carpenter has argued:

> Within the dominant empiricist approach are half-buried value assumptions which need to be prised out and exposed to the light of day. One of these is that nursing history is the history of general hospital nursing. Other branches receive scanty, if any, attention. In this way historians confirm, rather than question, the dominance of hospital nursing in the constellation of nursing and nursing-linked occupations.[9]

This view is shared by a group of radical nurses based in Boston, Massachussetts.[10] They argue that the emphasis which nurses place on professionalisation and professionalism, seen in a nursing history which is the history of the reform of general hospital nursing and which therefore focuses on what Carpenter calls 'the politics of reform and the lives and activities of nursing reformers',[11] leads to a 'carrot and stick' situation. The drive to become a profession, to develop those attributes which Cynthia Woods rehearses here in Chapter 10, and to get the carrots which professional status promises — 'increased respect, rewards, and supposed improvement'[12] — may have been at the expense of the very qualities which delineate nursing, in particular, the stewardship of the 'patient's dignity and over-all well-being'.[13]

4

Ruth Hawker, in her contribution, looks at the historical dimensions of this exchange — nursing professionalism for a patient-centred approach to caring. The Boston Nurses Group argues that in that exchange, nurses have lost out to administrators — lay and nursing — neither of whom share their world views. The emphasis on developing professionalism, in which nurses are taught that they are 'unique and better than other health care workers', 'can be used to exploit nurses'.[14]

But historians are surely correct when they dissect the processes of professionalisation in order to understand how it was that independence gave way to subservience, dependency and exploitation.[15] In so doing they do not merely expose the power struggles which characterise nursing's past but also point towards a future in which nursing professionalism equates with autonomy. Historical interest in professionalism should obviate a repetition of precisely those situations against which Carpenter, Hawker and the Boston Nurses Group warn. Sidney Krampitz, in her chapter 'Nursing Power and Nursing Politics' makes that point forcibly.

So there is here no apology for including at least four chapters which directly address professionalisation from an historical perspective. It is not simply a fascination with and acceptance of the supremacy of general nursing and general hospital nursing, although it would be a misreading of history not to see that that was precisely what happened. Nursing history, in subjecting the processes by which general nursing achieved its occupational supremacy to critical study, uncovers a wealth of material about those other groups and organisations which lost the struggle. The new history of nursing, which Celia Davies was confident would emerge, has done so in these essays.

If professionalisation is the linking theme of the papers in this volume, each treats the subject in different ways. Readers familiar with general sociological approaches to professionalisation will find Woods's article an interesting rehearsal of the issues within nursing. Her argument, that nursing professionalised at the expense of autonomy, finds an echo, as we have already noted, in Ruth Hawker's contribution. However, Hawker has more to say than nurses lost their autonomy as the hospital system developed. She is concerned with the consequences of professionalisation — by doctors and nurses — on their 'clients' — the patients and their families. In her chapter she suggests that the needs of these two developing professions were met within the institution, the hospital, and that the rules and codes of behaviour which the institution formulated served to discipline both the patients and the professionals, perhaps to the detriment of both.

In my own contribution I take up Hawker's theme about the power of the institution over those working in or using it. There I argue that the metaphor of the 'firm' — familiar to nurses, doctors, patients and watchers of TV and films — was rooted in reality. The hospital operated as a business enterprise even when it was a public, i.e. state-controlled, organisation. The profit and loss accounting methods inevitably engulfed the nurses, so that they became part of the 'costs' of the institution, to be paid for out of fragile revenues. What little autonomy the institutional nurse had was soon lost to the need of the hospital to keep its books balanced.

The loss of autonomy, which many of the contributors see as consequent to the drive to professionalise at almost any cost, is examined from a different perspective in Alice Friedman's chapter. Hannah Porn was an independent midwife, working with apparent success in Boston, Massachusetts. Her very success was like a red rag to those medical men who were seeking to medicalise childbirth and thus to exclude women from the practice of midwifery. Friedman chronicles the attempts by some of the Boston medical fraternity to outlaw Hannah Porn and her fellow workers; that campaign was successful and Hannah spent a considerable period in prison for her activities. Readers familiar with the work of Jean Donnison in England and that of Ehrenreich and English in the United States will sympathise with Friedman's analysis of this blatant example of sexual politics and power relations.[16]

Laura Linebach also shows that outside the hospitals and general nursing, groups of nurses were able to maintain their autonomy whilst evolving and extending their professional role. We are still waiting for a scholarly account of district and home nursing in Great Britain, although both Monica Baly (who contributes a paper to this volume on the Nightingale nurses) and Anne Summers at the Wellcome Unit for the History of Medicine are currently working in this area. Linebach's case study from Kansas City helps to fill in some of the gaps, and at the same time demonstrates the importance of local studies in the history of nursing. Her introduction also suggests that the careful addition of a fictional portrait can enhance historical scholarship.

In her contribution, Olga Maranjian Church looks at another area of non-general nursing, asylum or mental nursing. She charts the development of the mental nurse from the early years of the asylum; through the medicalisation of what may have been in essence social stresses; the intervention by general medicine and nursing into the field of psychiatry and psychiatric hospitals; to recent changes where the emphasis has switched from mental illness to mental health. The nurse's role in mental health maintenance and in mental health is a fairly recent development and one which has yet to occur in the general field.

Finally, three authors look at the Nightingale phenomenon. Monica Baly, drawing on her recently published account of the early years of the Nightingale Fund, looks closely at whether the experiment worked or was even fully tried. She shows how transient was Nightingale's own interest and involvement in the school and rescues Henry Bonham Carter from relative obscurity to put him clearly centre stage in that period in nursing's history. Krampitz takes a similar theme: she examines the Yale experiment in nurse training which drew heavily upon the perceived Nightingale schema. Both are clear that each was an experiment which, for a variety of reasons, did not entirely match any plan which Nightingale herself might have proposed. Josephine Castle provides us with a similar story as well as opening up to a wider audience the ways in which nursing in Australia differs from its original model, England and Nightingale. The current move to an all-graduate entry to nursing in Australia, reflecting similar concerns in the United States, will have significance for British nurses, particularly in the light of the recently published report on nurse education, *Project 2000*.

Two points should be made by way of conclusion. First, Carpenter is clearly mistaken in his attempt to relegate the history of nursing to a chapter in labour history. Putting aside the niceties of academic disciplines, there is more to nursing history than labour history has so far demonstrated itself able to discuss, not least in that nursing involves women as skilled workers. Second, there is a certain universality about the contributions presented here. That is not just the result of the selection process or because they deal with similar themes and problems. The peculiarities of the nineteenth century — which included economic, political and social imperial expansion by the industrialised nations of Europe and America which gave rise to the specific nineteenth-century characteristics of modern nursing —

7

produced similar tensions and stresses within those societies touched by that expansion. However, as the book as a whole shows, each developed different strategies to overcome those difficulties and with varying degrees of success.

NOTES

1. Celia Davies (ed.), *Rewriting nursing history* (Croom Helm, London, 1981), p.9.

2. Christopher Maggs,'Nursing history as historiography' in *New perspectives in nursing history: papers presented at a forum, 10 September 1982* (King's Fund Centre, London, 1982).

3. Mick Carpenter, 'Asylum nursing before 1914: a chapter in the history of labour' in Davies (ed.), *Rewriting nursing history*, p.125.

4. Carpenter, 'Asylum nursing before 1914', p.125.

5. This point is discussed by Katherine Williams, 'From Sarah Gamp to Florence Nightingale: a critical study of hospital nursing systems from 1840 to 1897' in Davies (ed.), *Rewriting nursing history*.

6. Celia Davies, 'Introduction: the contemporary challenge in nursing history' in Davies (ed.), *Rewriting nursing history*, p.11.

7. Williams, 'From Sarah Gamp to Florence Nightingale', pp.42–53.

8. Ibid., p.53.

9. Carpenter, 'Asylum nursing before 1914', p. 124.

10. Boston Nurses Group, *The false promise: professionalism in nursing* (New England Free Press, Somerville, Mass., 1978).

11. Carpenter, 'Asylum nursing before 1914', p.124.

12. Boston Nurses Group, *The false promise*, p.1.

13. Ibid., p.2.

14. Ibid., p.1.

15. Christopher Maggs, *Origins of general nursing* (Croom Helm, London, 1983), pp.173–4.

16. Jean Donnison, *Midwives and medical men: a history of inter-professional rivalries and women's rights* (Heinemann, London, 1977); B. Ehrenreich and D. English, *Complaints and disorders: the sexual politics of sickness* (Writers and Readers Publishing Co-operative, London, 1977, originally published 1973).

2

The Development of Professional Nursing in New South Wales, Australia

Josephine Castle

This chapter examines the development of nursing in New South Wales since 1900. The outline of change is familiar to historians of nursing: the gradual erosion of Nightingale precepts and practices and the emergence of a modern white-collar profession. But the process of change in New South Wales depended on a particular pattern of state intervention which directly influenced training within the hospitals and ultimately removed it from them, and indirectly through the arbitration system which enabled nurses more easily to compare themselves with other workers.

Nursing proved more resistant to change than other white-collar occupations because of its unique system of training and the work process which this entailed. The living-in requirement meant a thorough integration of working and non-working life making ward discipline and the protocol of rank automatic responses for most trainees. The greatest obstacle to change was the apprenticeship system of training, which in nursing persisted long after other skilled and semi-skilled occupations transferred the burden of training to the formal education institutions of the state. In relation to these occupations nursing changed from a relatively well-paid female occupation to become, in the 1950s, a less well-paid one where the skills failed to keep pace with the higher educational standards of the community at large. But at the same time changes in medical technology and the pattern of disease meant that greater professional skill was required.

The profession responded by lifting entry and training standards. Work in the wards changed as nurses aides took over 'housekeeping' tasks. But impetus from within the profession was not sufficient to break the Nightingale mould and training

9

remained 'on the job'. This reduced the professional status and pay of nurses leading to dissatisfaction and ultimately to militancy.

This paper looks at the interaction of the nursing profession and the state over 80 years leading to the transfer of nurse training out of hospitals and into the advanced education sector. Nursing in New South Wales was the last of the paramedical specialities to cast off the apprenticeship system. By removing basic education from hospitals to the advanced education sector and establishing a wide range of postgraduate courses, educational standards in nursing have risen substantially. But they did not keep pace with the general rise in educational standards for the Australian workforce as a whole, nor with standards in other paramedical fields such as physiotherapy or radiography, or in other white-collar jobs like teaching. This long process of change has, in Australia as elsewhere, involved the intervention of the state. Each Australian state had passed Registration Acts for nurses by 1930 and in each state before the Second World War nurses came under the jurisdiction of Arbitration Courts or Wages Boards. The Australasian Trained Nurses' Association (ATNA) formed in New South Wales in 1899 established branches in other states, encouraging a national similarity in standards of training. In each state the centralising tendencies of governments also operated to minimise regional differences and create uniformity on a national scale. The focus of this paper is on New South Wales, but for the reasons outlined, the uniformity of development between states means that the history of nursing in one state is a good general introduction to national trends.

Australian nursing has always had close links with government. A hospital was founded by Governor Phillip soon after the arrival of the First Fleet in 1778. In 1868 government initiative and funds brought six Nightingale nurses to New South Wales to reform the Sydney Infirmary and to set up a training school there from which trained nurses would graduate and move to other hospitals all over New South Wales, thus lifting standards everywhere.[2] Such direct intervention in the labour market was in keeping with the entrepreneurial role of the state in colonial Australia.

By 1899 nurses in New South Wales were sufficiently numerous and collectively self-conscious to form an association, the ATNA. Its primary object was to secure professional recognition and training for nurses by stringent self-regulation. The

ATNA began a register of trained nurses, authorised a curriculum of training and laid down minimum standards for hospitals wishing to qualify as certified training schools. It lobbied the state government to withhold subsidy from hospitals using nursing staff not on the ATNA register and began a campaign for a state Registration Act.[3] The Act was passed in 1924 and established a Nurses' Registration Board which continued the practices sanctioned by the ATNA. For example, the minimum training period of three years, varying to four or five according to the amount of clinical experience, recommended by the ATNA in 1903, now became statutory.

But all of this was done with initiative and guidance from doctors. It was the doctors who encouraged the formation of the ATNA. Its first president was Dr Norton Manning. Four of five executive members of the first committee were male doctors and they provided five of the nine ordinary committee members.[4] Resolutions adopted in 1916 provided that one-fifth of the governing council of the ATNA be 'duly qualified medical practitioners' (who were, in practice, almost certain to be male). The Registration Act itself, first introduced into Parliament in 1913, was delayed for a decade because of the refusal of some doctors to have nurses on the Board.[5] Nurses were guaranteed just over half, i.e. 13, out of 25 positions on the Council. Medical dominance of the ATNA declined after the Registration Act, though representation continued. But the dominance was transferred to the new Nurses' Registration Board, which replaced the ATNA as the foremost regulatory body. Under the new Act four out of seven members were to be doctors.

Such preponderance at statutory levels was paralleled in the hospital training schools where doctors played the primary role in the education of nurses until the 1950s or 1960s. Theoretical training in medical and surgical nursing was in New South Wales provided by medical practitioners. In metropolitan hospitals lectures for nurses were given by the honoraries (consultants), specialists in a particular field.[6] Country hospitals co-opted local general practitioners.[7] Matrons lectured on ethics and general nursing,[8] as well as organising and administering the whole training programme. There were no nurse educators specifically designated as such before the 1930s. In 1935 Royal Prince Alfred Hospital appointed a sister tutor.[9] In 1948 the *Australian Nurses' Journal* (ANJ) noted that 'less than 36 training schools' had sister tutors and that 'only 6 or 7 of these hold University qualifications or have had special training as nurse teachers'.[10]

Thus before the Second World War, nursing was essentially a practical training acquired almost wholly on the job with a small theoretical component 'just fitted in'. The resource implications were minimal. There were no schools in the sense of formal institutions totally committed to learning with a staff of teachers and a set of pupils. After 1945 there was a greater investment of resources in time and personnel. Tutor sisters appeared in most hospitals[11] and, with the establishment of preliminary training schools, some hospital time, as distinct from nurses' own time, was earmarked for the formal training of nurses.[12] Thereafter the formal aspects of training grew in importance. More specialised staff appeared whose sole function was teaching and not ward duties or administration. Nurse education thus began, belatedly, to command its own resources.

Before these developments the training of nurses by matrons, ward sisters and doctors was virtually without extra cost. Hospitals provided the educators from their existing staff. Matrons and doctors did double duty as theoreticians and practitioners and, perhaps the most essential feature, the trainee nurses doubled as workers. The hospital system depended on this constantly renewable source of cheap labour.

Trainees before 1953 in New South Wales were required to have 78 hours of formal instruction as a minimum; in practice most hospitals stuck to this minimum, while requiring nurses to train for four years which exceeded the minimum. Lectures covered anatomy, physiology, medical, surgical and general nursing, hygiene and infection and invalid cookery.[13] They were generally 'fitted in' in off duty time. In some small hospitals the lectures were scheduled without regard for nurses' on or off duty times. One 1930s trainee wrote:

The nursing lectures were given by the doctors at their convenience and were consequently given at the oddest of times; one had to find a replacement from off duty, if one happened to be on duty; this seemed to work out as, if unwilling, when her time [for lectures] came she would find unwillingness and have to miss her lecture.[14]

The 'reliever' had to be roughly equivalent in experience and acceptable to the ward sister, which made the trainee's job even harder. Thus did the hospitals, and indirectly the state, transfer much of the cost of education to the nurses — who paid for it with their off duty time, or if on duty with substitutes and a 'pay back' scheme operated by nurses themselves. In bigger metropolitan hospitals with large intakes of trainees, lectures were scheduled more systematically and occurred in off duty time. In all hospitals those off duty, but away from the hospital, had to return for lectures. Final examinations were taken in off duty time. Most of the financial burden of formal training was thus borne by nurses.

The establishment of preliminary training schools committed hospital time to training in ward practice. The logical correlate of this was the block system for instruction in the theoretical syllabus where nurses devoted all their on duty time to theory lectures and examinations; doing their ward work in stretches in between throughout their training. Such a system allowed trainees to give their undivided attention to theory and to come to lectures freed from the physical strain of ward duties. It was recommended for New South Wales hospitals as early as 1943[15] but not implemented until the 1960s.

In 1967 most hospitals in New South Wales moved from a requirement of four years practical training to three years. Significantly, it was about this time that they began taking enrolled nursing aides to compensate for the lost year of trainee labour. By this time also, the formal component of training had risen to 1,000 hours; it reached 1,200 by 1979. Thus a three-year trained nurse graduating in 1970 had more than ten times the amount of formal theoretical training compared with a four-year trained nurse graduating in 1940. The proportion of theoretical training to practical in 1970 was more than one-third, in 1940, it was perhaps one-thirtieth.

What brings about change of this magnitude? In general terms it is one of the social consequences wrought by sustained growth in the national income and full employment after 1940. An economy growing in complexity demands more and more tertiary services, especially in health. Demands are generated from within and without the health services for more, better and different services. Government funding, inquiry and reform usually proceeded hand-in-hand with the professional associations who were also responding to perceived deficiencies in the health system which were apparent in the hospital wards.

Beginning in the war years, a series of enquiries articulated the deficiencies of nurse education in a changing society. The first of these was the *Kelly Report* of 1943 in New South Wales which looked at nurse training in the light of the war-time shortage and recommended a three-year training scheme, a block system and preliminary training schools. The enquiry was assisted in its task by the ATNA who supported the criticism of the paucity of theoretical training then evident. Both the state government and the ATNA were concerned at the loss of potential nurses to more lucrative occupations during the war and the likelihood that losses would continue in the postwar period, in view of predictions for the continuance of full employment. These problems would be compounded by the postwar plans for the expansion of health services expressed in the Social Services Act of 1946. Many more graduate nurses would be wanted, warned the ATNA in 1948.[16]

In 1949 the ATNA, the New South Wales Nurses' Association, the Institute of Hospital Matrons and trained nurses from Canberra, set up a college of nursing for postgraduate teaching of nurses in such areas as administration and industrial nursing. Before 1949 the only postgraduate nursing courses offered in New South Wales were in obstetrics and psychiatry. But the college was without government funding for the next decade and student paid fees to cover administrative costs. The supervisory, clerical and most lecturing staff donated their services. Various hospitals provided lecture rooms.[17]

During the 1960s over-full employment made recruitment even more difficult and provoked further professional soul-searching. The Institute of Hospital Matrons of New South Wales reported in 1967 that:

> emphasis has been placed during training on nursing procedures in order to prepare a nurse as quickly as possible for ward duties without producing the necessary correlated theoretical instruction. This has resulted in the production of a nurse who is restricted in outlook, resistant to change and unable to cope confidently with the scientific and technical advances in medicine and the social problems of nurses.[18]

But old habits die hard and the matrons could not bring themselves to sever the nexus between education and employment. They recommended that schools of nursing be established each associated with a group of hospitals[19] and it was left to experts outside the profession, the Truskett Committee, to recommend to the New South Wales Parliament in 1970 that nursing be made part of the tertiary education system. This was echoed at Federal level by the *Report on Nurse Education and Training* in 1978, which recommended that: '. . . the preparation of nurses remains one of the major areas of vocational education which has not been substantially integrated within the general post-secondary system'. The report argued that hospitals alone could not provide educational experience for nurse trainees: 'which would enlarge their vision, develop their potential resources and make them aware of the social, political and cultural problems they must face as citizens'.[20]

The change in attitude represented here was already firmly registered in New South Wales, where in 1977 responsibility for the training of nurses was transferred from the Minister of Health to the Minister for Education.[19] Nursing education was placed in the advanced education sector: at first colleges of advanced education offered associate diplomas and then the universities offered diplomas. Training schools based in individual hospitals were closed and staff transferred to regional schools and thence to the advanced education sector. Thus, over a century, the training of nurses moved from being cheap, haphazard and essentially practical to a training which is expensive, systematic and increasingly theoretical.

Much of the Nightingale system[21] had been modified or eradicated over the span of a century. The nexus between work and training was almost gone. Matron's authority over training and morals was no longer supreme. Trainees no longer lived in as a matter of compulsion. Theory bulked much larger in their lives. Perhaps most importantly these changes altered the nurse-doctor relationship — nurses no longer accepted handmaiden status. In the 1970s feminist attacks on patriarchy brought questions of male dominance uncomfortably to the fore. Some nurses applied the insights of feminist theory to their profession as did many academics who were beginning to examine nursing.[22] But in the work done by nurses feminist insights were but slowly reflected.

While work and training were synonymous, work relationships and the job itself were unlikely to change. In New South Wales trainee nurses were primarily workers, for the whole period while hospital-based training schools existed. Training was offered in exchange for cheap and plentiful labour, yet nurses from the beginnings of the Nightingale system had trouble identifying themselves as workers. Ideals of service, dedication and vocation made, and for some still make, an obfuscating

15

ideology which inhibits a realisation of their material circumstances. There are three possible explanations: the bourgeois origins of many nurses, the nature of the work process on the wards and the system of living in.

A large proportion of the recruits and especially of those occupying higher administrative positions were middle class. Nursing was reformed and reshaped by Florence Nightingale specifically as a suitable occupation for middle-class women.[23] She established her training school in 1860, four years after the formation of the Society for Promoting the Employment of Women and at a time when the problem of the 'surplus women' (of the middle classes) was a subject of much topical concern. Some reformers tried to improve the standard of education for middle-class girls to make them employable as governesses.[24] The Middle Class Emigration Society preached emigration to the colonies as the solution. There were few occupations available to middle-class young ladies without husband or father to support them.

Nursing appeared as one solution for those waiting to marry or for those destined never to marry. Thus nursing began its modern existence typed as an occupation suitable for respectable middle-class girls, and thereafter in both Britain and the colonies attracted recruits from this class. This provided a solid base from which to develop an idealistic view. In twentieth-century New South Wales nursing continued to attract girls from well-off backgrounds as well as recruits from the working class.

A second explanation is that there may be something in the nature of the work process itself which inhibits the self-perception of nurses. What is the nature of the work done by nurses? How does it relate to the requirements of living-in? And what changes have taken place in the last two or three decades which seem to have facilitated the process of identification of nursing as work, or as a job like other jobs?

The work of nurses has always been complex and varied, demanding a combination of practical skill, manual dexterity and intelligence with caring. Duties include domestic tasks, general patient care, healing functions, observations and tests and, for senior nurses and sisters, the instruction of juniors. The proportion of these duties within the total work of nurses has changed over time. Nurses in the 1980s compared with nurses in the 1920s, do very little domestic work, but a great many tests and observations requiring the use of sophisticated machinery and equipment.

Nursing procedures have obviously changed greatly in response to changes in medical knowledge. For example, medical wards in the 1920s and 1930s contained many patients with nephritis or in diabetic comas. New discoveries like insulin and antibiotics have changed all this. In the 1920s even small hospitals had about half a dozen cases of typhoid per year.[25] Typhoid cases required intensive nursing and much heavy lifting as the current orthodoxy banned movement so as to minimise the risk of haemorrhage or perforation.

In the early years of the century nurses were looking after patients in an all-inclusive way. Patients were kept much longer in bed; some were not allowed to move without assistance; hospital stays were much longer. Nurses not only buttered bread, counted cutlery and stoked fires; they sterilized their own equipment, made up swabs and splints and rolled bandages. Now rapid mobility after surgery has eliminated much heavy lifting and full sponging. Gone are the days of spika bandages and complete immobility for hernia repair cases. The care and use of equipment has been revolutionised by the advent of plastic disposable needles, syringes and tubes. Even the humble bedpan appears in plastic these days.

Nursing work has always been defined in relation to the work of other workers involved in patient care, most obviously and importantly in relation to the work of doctors, but also in relation to domestics, clerks and, in the twentieth century, paramedics like physiotherapists and radiographers.[26] At some hospitals, at certain periods nurses as a matter of course have provided physiotherapy for patients, taken x-rays, recorded case histories, swept floors, made up swabs and splints or special diets and cooked and served meals.[27] The trend in hospitals since 1945 has been for these functions to be performed by specialists, i.e. non-nurses. Most hospitals now employ ward clerks to take case histories, and do other paper work. Kitchen staff now cook and serve meals. Domestics do all the sweeping and cleaning of floors. Radiographers have their own special department as do physiotherapists in even the smallest hospitals.

But the functions are still not entirely clear cut. Nursing is a 24-hour activity, clerking is not, nor cleaning, nor physiotherapy. Patients are unlikely to require physiotherapy at midnight, but they may well vomit on the ward floor; and hygiene demands that vomit be cleaned up — by nurses. After hours admissions must be processed and case histories taken — such clerical work must be done by nurses. What work then specifically defines a nurse?

During hospital-based training a nurse working on the wards did all types of work, but there was a complex division of labour based on seniority. Thus junior trainees did domestic duties, making beds, emptying pans and urinals and arranging flowers, while senior nurses were responsible for the healing functions like dressings and injections. Sisters and senior nurses shared the task of training juniors. This division of labour endured on the wards for most of the period to 1980. The decline in the availability of trainees has meant that nurses' aides or nurses' assistants now do most of the domestic work and some basic patient care. Experiments such as task or patient assignment also alter this basic division of labour, but these processes have not been widely adopted.[28]

At Wollongong Hospital in the mid-1960s the division of labour on a surgical ward was this: the senior nurses did all the more complicated treatment jobs like fluid balances, drains, sutures and putting up intravenous drips. They would do dressings and teach the others as they did so. A senior would be responsible for making sure that those junior to her got morning and afternoon tea. A third year nurse would do mixtures and pills. A second year or late first year would do the leftovers. The most junior first year would be allocated pans, blowers, beds and serving patients' meals. Everyone might do a little of the beds and washes. Fourth year nurses had to weigh out special diets, e.g. for diabetics. Now these come ready packaged from the kitchen made up according to instructions from the hospital's dietitian.[29]

Cleaning bulked large in the lives of nurse trainees at this small country hospital in New South Wales in the 1920s and 1930s. Most of them, when asked what they remembered most about their training, said 'cleaning'. Trainees of the 1960s reported fewer domestic tasks. Rituals like throwing moist tea leaves on the floors to lay the dust do not feature in their reports, but the 'ward tidy' before visiting hours endured from the 1920s to the 1980s. It was a strenuous half-hour twice daily falling mainly to the junior nurses and involved wiping lockers, changing paper rubbish bags, straightening bedding and filling patients' water jugs.

The Arbitration Commission of New South Wales registered

this important change in the domestic content of nursing work in the Award of 1953 which said:

> nurses, student nurses, nursing aides . . . shall not be required to perform as a matter of routine, the following duties viz. washing, sweeping, polishing and/or dusting of floors, walls or windows of wards . . . [except] in an isolation block or where the performance of those duties involves disinfection . . . and [except] . . . during the first thirteen weeks of training . . .[30]

It is doubtful whether nurses training in the 1980s would agree with the trainee nurse of 1947 who maintained that 'to be a good nurse you have to be a good housekeeper'.[31] But other functions endured. Despite the trend to early ambulation patients still needed pans and urinals and these needed to be emptied and washed. Nurses whether starting in the 1920s or the 1970s recalled that in the first year of training they saw more of the pan room than anything else.[32] As nurses progressed through their training other duties were added.

Built into the work process was a complicated and tightly integrated hierarchy. At the pinnacle were honoraries (consultants). 'They are Gods and sisters are the right hand of God', commented one trainee of the late 1970s. Matron occupied a position only slightly less exalted than honoraries. Residents (interns) were fairly low on the scale but the fact that they were doctors gave them, in theory, a superior status. In practice, many nurses were irritated by this and by the residents' lack of practical skills.[33] But it was amongst nurses themselves that the seniority system was most entrenched. For example, a trainee was senior to another in the same year if she preceded her into the hospital by as much as a single day. First years stood back to allow second years to precede them through doorways. Seniors had first turn at the tea trolley and so on. One nurse (1934) recounted this experience:

> . . . I was called by a senior nurse to go to her in the middle of the ward. She was one none of us liked working under, and she made me go back to the end of the ward and walk up to her, head erect and hands behind my back in front of all the patients. This was a means of putting one in one's place.[34]

And these experiences persisted well into the postwar period. A trainee of the 1950s said the juniors were 'menials, like ants' and another (1966) said that 'the seniority system tramples you; when you first kick off you are told you are nothing'. The system was inbuilt and self-validating for those juniors became seniors and took up their positions of command in the hierarchy. Respect given in early years was paid back in later ones. In the 1980s junior nurses are still required to stand respectfully with hands behind the back when speaking to seniors. All nurses interviewed pointed to rules and restrictions, which by their existence denied the fact that on the ward they were expected to be responsible adults carrying out life-saving procedures.[35]

The protocol of rank even governed off duty friendships. When trainees lived in, it was almost mandatory that these be formed with people from the same year.[36] Discipline and rank were built into the life of nurses in the nurses' home. Living in was a central experience for nurses in New South Wales (and elsewhere) until the end of the 1970s. But the decline of hospital-based training schools and the revolution in training has brought to an end the system of compulsory living in. Arguably it is this change which has most contributed to changes in nurses' perception of themselves and to the decline of the Nightingale system.

In few other occupations was living in an integral part of the work experience. It was the main cause of that sense of separation from other workers experienced by nurses. Analogies drawn from religious experience — the cloister, the ghetto — are frequently employed to describe the system, and with some justice. Before the Second World War when nurses had one day off per week, and two to four weeks annual leave, a nurse was almost literally dedicated to the workplace. Off duty time was often spent in the nurses' home because of the vagaries of shifts and rosters. Night nurses were required to sleep in at the home during the day and leisure time was spent with other nurses, by choice and necessity — for who else kept such hours? Time off rarely coincided with weekends when the rest of the workforce was free. Broken shifts (a common feature at many New South Wales hospitals till the 1940s) made it even more difficult for nurses to make use of off duty time. 'Passes' were required for leaving the home[37] to visit the outside world. These were limited and there were strict curfews. Non-compliance was severely punished and frequent offences brought disgrace and dismissal.

By the 1960s nurses had more time off (two days per week),

more annual leave, and leave passes were more readily obtained. By the end of the 1960s the live in requirements were sometimes waived, senior nurses were allowed to 'live out' and the system was much less rigid. By 1980 the living in requirement at Wollongong Hospital had been reduced to three months. Married trainees were now commonplace, whereas before the war marriage was barred, if not officially then effectively, by the living in requirements. Nurses in the 1980s are much more like other workers. For example, the attitude to overtime has changed greatly. It is possible to trace the evolution of the reformed attitude in trainees at Wollongong Hospital from the 1930s to the 1980s.

In the 1930s no nurse was permitted to depart from ward duty until she could report to the ward sister 'all work complete, may I leave now?' Matron told one nurse (1936) on her first day 'No overtime is paid at this hospital. There is never too much work to do, there are only incompetent nurses.'[38] Overtime was worked every day since the de facto starting and finishing times for shifts were as much as one hour before or after the official time. Such de facto hours were observed until the 1960s. Officially, day shift ran from 6.30 a.m. to 2.30 p.m. Half an hour was allowed for lunch. Morning and afternoon tea were not strict entitlements, and if taken never exceeded 10 minutes. All nurses accepted this unwritten rule 'otherwise you couldn't get through all the work', since breakfast at 7.45 a.m. took at least 20 minutes and matron's rounds were at 10.00 a.m. by which time all the beds had to be made and patients washed and tidied. A 1950 trainee never remembers starting later than 5.00 a.m. as a junior. But 'as a senior one could get away with being a little later' say about 5.45 a.m. if a 'light' day was expected. The early start was still in force in 1971, though it had by then dwindled to about 15 minutes, making a 6.15 a.m. start for juniors on a 6.30 shift.[39]

Shifts did not end at the official time either. If a new case was admitted at 2.28 p.m. then the day shift staff were responsible and stayed until the patient was fully admitted. Ambulance officers could sometimes be persuaded to keep cases in the corridor for an extra few minutes until the next shift officially began. After the war the concept of paid overtime slowly won acceptance. A trainee (1957) remembers that: 'Whether you got overtime — it depended on Sister — if she thought you'd been working flat out all day she would sign; otherwise not.'

Another trainee of the 1950s recalls that it had to be at least 30 minutes over or it could not be claimed. But every day, nurses still worked unpaid overtime.

> On morning duty we used to go on at half past five instead of half past six . . . we only used to go on that hour earlier to get everybody sponged; we wanted that all done before breakfast. About the end of my third year there — they brought it in . . . must have been the union . . . stepped in . . . and they said 'no you must not go on at half past six'. But we used to hate it, because . . . after [the nurses'] breakfast, the doctors would be coming and there'd be patients all around that weren't washed; their beds weren't made, they weren't even in clean clothes . . . and you used to like your ward clean and spotless and really up and on the knocker, everything right for when doctors came and Matron used to do rounds about 9.00 o'clock, too . . . and you wanted the ward right. It never seemed the same to me when the patients weren't sitting up nice and clean and everything done by breakfast time.[40]

Thus did pride in good work override industrial considerations of payment for actual hours worked. But this was in line with an ambivalence which most nurses felt about nursing. From the first trainees to the last, the nurses interviewed maintained that for them nursing was more than a job — if they had wanted just a job there were easier ways to earn a living and for more money; most of them came into nursing because they wanted to help people, or because they thought it would be an interesting job where you could do things and move around, not like an office job.[41] It is easy to see therefore how unwritten conventions about unpaid overtime became established and passed unchallenged for many years. This special approach to their work colours attitudes to such important issues as pay and unionisation.

Nursing like other female occupations has traditionally meant low pay and long hours. In 1907 the Commonwealth Arbitration Court fixed a basic wage a standard based on the needs of an average unskilled male with four dependants, a wife and three children. For 60 years this concept of the family wage, taking as its standard the adult male breadwinner, dominated wage determination in Australia. The female basic wage took the single unmarried female without dependants as its standard and was fixed at approximately 54 per cent of the male rate until 1950, when it was raised to 75 per cent. While the concept of the family wage prevailed female wages were held down. It was not until the abolition of the concept of the basic wage and its replacement by the total wage in 1967 that the Arbitration Commission moved away from the concept of the family wage embodied in the Harvester judgement of 1907.[42] This cleared the way for the equal pay judgements of 1969 and 1974 which in turn helped to lift wages in nursing and other female occupations.[43]

As Table 2.1 shows, in the 1930s nurses' pay was better than female pay in other occupations. In New South Wales in October 1936 the basic wage for an adult female was $3.80.[42] The award for first and second year trainees was less, based on the probability that nearly all first and second years would be juveniles i.e. less than 20 years of age, since entrants to nursing were required to be 18 years of age. The award stipulated that no adult trainee could be paid less than the basic wage.

Final year trainees were awarded $5.00 weekly, better than the average weekly wage for adult females which was $4.57 at the end of 1936. But against this must be set the fact of longer hours in nursing, the lack of overtime and penalty rates and the fact that nurses were older than other female workers who entered the workforce at 14. The number of hours constituting a full week's work varied between occupations, but average working hours for females in 1936 were 43.93 and the average hourly rate was 10-1/2c.[44] But trainees and assistants in nursing worked a 52-hour week on day shifts; so their hourly rate was less, e.g. 9-1/2c. per hour for final year trainees. Hours were longer still for those on night duty: 55 including meal times. Moreover trainee nurses were required to live-in and pay board — usually $2.00 weekly (this was the maximum). Therefore their take-home pay was less.

In 1936 the pay of trained nurses reflected their skill and training. Staff nurses were paid $6.75 a week, about 50 per cent more than the average weekly female wage but less than the basic wage for an unskilled adult male ($7.00 in October 1936). Sisters in their first year of service were paid $7.50 weekly, $8.00 in second year and $8.50 thereafter.

In New South Wales at the end of 1953 the basic wage for adult females was $18.05. The award for a first year trainee was $14.75 — 85 per cent of the basic wage, about the same as in 1936. Final year trainees were awarded 25c less than the basic wage, whereas in 1936 they earned $1.20 or about 34 per cent more. Thus wages in nursing in comparison with other female occupations seem

Table 2.1: A comparison of wages in nursing in NSW 1936-81 with female average award wages

NSW public hospital nurses' award salaries per week (general nursing)	1936 $	1953 $	1973 $	1981 $
First year trainee	3.25	14.75	42.30	169.10
(% Female average award wages [FAW])	(71.3)	(74.3)	(62.8)	(82.8)
Final year trainee	5.00	17.75	61.80	208.50
(% FAW)	(109.6)	(89.5)	(91.8)	(102.2)
Registered Nurse: first year out	6.75	23.45	82.90	242.60
(% FAW)	(148.0)	(119.2)	(123.1)	(118.8)
Registered nurse: fifth year out or equivalent	8.50	25.95	98.40	279.60
(% FAW)	(186.4)	(130.8)	(146.1)	(137.0)
NSW				
Female average award wages (adult workers excluding overtime)	4.56	19.84	67.33	204.09

Table 2.2: Weekly hours of labour: nurses' award and all adult female workers

NSW	1936	1953	1973
Trainees (all years)	52	40	40
All registered nurses	48	40	40
All adult female workers: average hours (excluding overtime)	43.9	39.9	39.5

relatively worse in 1953 than in 1936. But it must be remembered that the basic wage had risen substantially to 75 per cent of the male rate in 1950 and that all workers, nurses included, by then officially worked a 40-hour week. But as Table 2.1 shows, nurses' wages expressed as a percentage of average female award wages are relatively worse for all categories except first year trainees. Registered nurses after five years' experience earned 131 per cent (rounded figures) of average female earnings in 1953 compared with 186 per cent in 1936. In 1973 these wages were better at 146 per cent of the average. First year trainees in 1973 were relatively worse off than in 1953 and 1936. As Table 2.3 shows, in 1953 nurses' earnings in relation to average weekly

Table 2.3: A comparison of nurses' wages with male average award wages

NSW	1936	1953	1973	1981
	$	$	$	$
1. Male average award wages (adult workers, excluding overtime)	8.55	29.67	78.13	209.73
2. Registered nurse: fifth year out (or equivalent)	8.50	25.95	98.40	279.60
(2 as percentage of 1)	(99.4)	(87.5)	(125.9)	(133.3)

Source: *Nurses' Awards* NSW 1936, 1953, 1973 and 1981.
Year Books of the Commonwealth of Australia nos. 33, 43, 64 and 67. Wages in 1936 & 1953 originally in shillings and pence have been converted to $A.

earnings for males were worse. In 1936 registered nurses with five years' experience earned only 5c. less than the average weekly earnings for males, in 1953 they earned $3.61 less. In 1973 their pay is much improved in relation to males and the upward trend is even greater in 1981.

In the 1980s there has been some improvement in wages as high staff turnover and shortages of nurses have caused pressure for wage rises. Even so, nurses were still relatively better off in the 1930s and despite the increased demands now made on nurses, their pay still fails to reflect their increased levels of skill and training.

After 1945 real wages rose generally, though more in some occupations than others. With full employment more of the trainees who had left school at 14 had been able to find jobs before entering the hospital at 17. They could therefore make comparisons with pay elsewhere, more easily than the recruits of the 1930s who found it more difficult, in a period of mass unemployment, to find jobs in the gap between leaving school and entering the hospital.

A male trainee (1978) had worked in the highly paid, largely male, occupation of accountancy before going nursing. He was earning $350 a week in 1978. As a first year trainee in that year he was paid $120 a week (and noted that a first year trainee teacher received $220). At graduation three years later his $230 was nowhere near his former salary (he calculates the opportunity cost of his training at $25,000). But in some ways this male nurse was much like the female recruits of the preceding 50 years. He really wanted to do nursing because it was interesting and satisfying and more than just a job. 'The people who thought of it as just a job, got weeded out — they could get $20 or $30 a week more working in a shop.' He attributed the poor pay and hours to nursing being a female occupation. Nurses' wages were either a single income or a second income, not a family wage and because of 'the Nightingale syndrome' nurses were not really prepared to fight for better pay and conditions.[48] Nurses had been listening for nearly a century to propaganda of this kind. In the 1930s an editorial from *The Times*, approvingly reprinted in the *ANJ*, asserted that:'. . . the profession of nursing cannot, and should not, compete for candidates against other professions, according to the ways of the market place. It will always be a calling apart — a service based on vocation, rather than on the hope of reward.'[49] A prominent Australian nurse reiterated these sentiments in 1948:

> . . . nursing is a special type of work and service . . . with human beings, not with the inanimate things, however important and valuable, dealt with in industry. At the same time it is just for this reason that the physical, psychological and emotional impacts on nurses are greater than workers in ordinary industry have to meet and that conditions for them must be improved if skilled nursing is to continue to exist.[50]

Nursing in relation to other female occupations looked less attractive in the period after 1945 than in prewar years. The long boom fed a seemingly limitless demand for female labour especially in the tertiary sector, but also in secondary industry. Female teachers in New South Wales achieved equal pay in 1958 and it was achieved in the public service after 1969. Overtime and penalty rates pushed up earnings. It was not until 1974 when the Commonwealth Arbitration Commission made its 'equal pay for work of equal value' judgement that nurses' pay improved considerably in relation to other female, and some male, occupations.

The conflict between vocation and poor conditions was emphasised in 1931 when nurses unwillingly entered the industrial arbitration system. In New South Wales during the 1920s industrial strife was intense and bitter and few workers were unaffected by it. At the time the main union in the field of health care was the Hospital Employees Association (HEA) founded in 1911 to cover employees in asylums, hospitals and the ambulance services.[51] By the mid-1920s it had achieved good coverage of asylums and ambulance services and covered domestics and miscellaneous staff of hospitals. It began, therefore, a campaign to recruit nurses. Organisers approached trainees at Sydney Hospital urging them to join the HEA and win an eight-hour day.[52] Some nurses began to complain about poor pay and conditions. The Sydney *Truth* published an anonymous article by a Sydney Hospital trainee criticising the conditions of training and in particular the despotic power of the matron.[53]

The Nurses' Registration Board set up in 1924, became the recipient of many industrial complaints and since it was not legally empowered to deal with industrial matters, the Board of Health appointed in 1929 seven 'supervisory' nurses to inspect hospitals throughout New South Wales.[54] Four of these inspectors with the blessing of the ATNA drafted rules for a nurses' association. The ATNA itself was not eligible to register as a trade union as it was not composed solely of employees. But there the matter rested until the HEA successfully applied to the New South Wales Arbitration Court for exclusive coverage of all health workers. In passing judgement Justice Piddington remarked that it was open to the nurses to form their own union, apply to the court for registration and remove themselves from the control of the HEA.[55]

But the nurses did not act until early 1931 when it appeared that the New South Wales government was about to legislate for compulsory unionism. This would have forced nurses to join the HEA, a body in which nurses would have only two out of nine council members. Therefore 'to preserve their professional identity' nurses met and decided to form the New South Wales Nurses' Association in April 1931 and seek registration as a trade union. The HEA lodged objections to this in the Arbitration Court. However, this did not affect the Association which officially became an industrial union in 1932 and obtained its first award in September 1936.[56]

From the account above it is obvious that many nurses were reluctant unionists and that even for those joining in 1931, it was largely a defensive measure against the HEA. When the ATNA polled its members seeking support for the new Association they witheld their endorsement, though only by a narrow majority.[57] Unionism posed ideological problems for nurses because of their belief in nursing as a special service demanding selfless dedication. Until 1930 the conflicts between service and industrial militancy were contained within the framework of the ATNA. The ATNA had proved adequate for the task of lobbying for state registration, standardising a training curriculum and in general working with doctors. But it was run by the upper echelons of the nursing and medical professions and was not concerned with wages, hours and living conditions for trainee nurses, or even the registered nurses who were beginning to indicate their discontent.

Registration as a trade union operating within an arbitration system did not solve their problems. It did help to standardise conditions among hospitals and ensured that nurses' wages were regularly adjusted for price changes under the system of quarterly cost of living adjustments which prevailed until 1953. It also placed an independent quasi-judicial body between the nurses and the direct influence of the state, which employed the majority of nurses and nurse trainees. But most importantly, it provided a mechanism which equated nurses with other workers in the determination of terms and conditions of employment.

The first award handed down by the Court in 1936 reflected existing conditions and was largely based on conditions in the larger public hospitals. But there were gains for the large number of nurses working outside public hospitals in the private sector either for themselves or in private hospitals. The Association was also successful in obtaining a preference in employment clause for unionists in this first award — an invaluable help to a new union struggling to establish itself.[58]

But the Nightingale philosophy and the training developed from it negated some basic union principles. Nurses are trained in self-abnegation, to place the welfare of patients first even if this means unpaid overtime and low wages. The logic of their ideals virtually *demand* poor pay and long hours as the outward and visible signs of the nurses' inward and spiritual vocation and devotion to patients. By extension it is easy to construct an argument that good nurses *cannot* be well paid and comfortably housed, because they would be 'in it for the money' and not the good of patients.

Thus the first edition of the *ANJ* explained that its object was 'to promote the interest of trained nurses in all matters affecting their work as a class'. The editorial asserted that this object was best served by establishing a system of registration and by ensuring minimum standards of training for nurses in New South Wales and by providing a forum for discussion. It was also important to provide nurses with a benefit scheme to support them while temporarily incapacitated. Thus straight industrial objectives were mingled with other more general ones, but the Association was clearly uneasy about these and was moved to defend itself:

. . . The Association is entitled to claim that it has so far carried out its work in no mere spirit of trades unionism and merely for the benefit of its members. In raising the standard of education amongst nurses and in publishing the Register . . . it has conferred benefits on the public both by providing for it, nurses better qualified to carry out the important duties of their calling and by enabling the public . . . to distinguish between those nurses who are qualified . . . and those nurses (so-called) who possess neither the training nor experience to render their employment safe or expedient . . .[59]

The New South Wales Nurses' Association was the direct heir of the ATNA in these attitudes. It was always an unwilling trade union. Amongst it objects at the end of 1981 were the promotion of industrial peace and efficiency; and to remain non-political and non-sectarian. Even for a white-collar union its stance was remarkably right of centre and far from militant. Yet nurses were becoming militant in the 1960s. In 1966 there were mass meetings and street marches in Sydney and country centres.[60] Subsequently when nurses went on strike, it was symbolic, unionists reported for duty out of uniform and patient care was not jeopardised. But strikes affecting patient care have begun to take place in the last two years and the transformation of nursing into an occupation much like any other seems complete.

Paradoxically in the 1980s when educational standards in nursing have never been higher, nursing offers poorer pay and conditions than many other white-collar jobs for women. This contrasts markedly with the 1930s when nursing as an occupation was comparatively well paid for both trainees and trained staff. As a skilled female occupation it ranked second only to teaching and even compared favourably with many male occupations. In 1936 a nursing sister with five years' experience earned only 5c. less than the average weekly award wage for males in New South Wales. By the 1950s nurses' pay was relatively lower in relation to average female wages in other occupations and was considerably worse than average male wages. In the 1970s and the 1980s the relativities have altered for the better but the relativities of 1936 have not been restored.

Nurses in the 1980s compare their pay and conditions with a much wider range of white-collar jobs than were available to women in prewar years. Female teachers, always at a comparative advantage, have streaked ahead since achieving equal pay with male teachers in 1958. Female public servants earn more than nurses as do the physiotherapists, radiographers and most medical technicians and social workers employed in their thousands by an expanding tertiary sector after the war. Full employment and rising real wages in the long postwar boom combined to create many more attractive job opportunities for women. Involvement in the arbitration system invites comparison with other workers. Internal pressures to change education and training assist the process. The motives for industrial militancy clearly exist.

Militancy grows as the decline of living in deprives the profession of opportunities to rebuild its cadre in the image of Nightingale. The end result is an occupation in the 1980s fundamentally altered from that created by Nightingale in the 1860s.

NOTES

1. E. Gamarnikow, 'Sexual division of labour: the case of nursing' in A. Kuhn and A. Wolpe (eds), *Feminism and materialism* (Routledge and Kegan Paul, London, 1978).

2. R. L. Russell, 'The training of nurses at the Lucy Osburn School of Nursing, Sydney Hospital 1868–1920', *Educational Enquiry*, vol. 2, part 1 (1979).

3. *Australasian Nurses' Journal* (AJN), vol.1, no.1 (March 1903), pp.1–3.

4. Ibid., p.5.

5. G. Law, 'I have never liked trade unionism' in E. Windschuttle (ed.), *Women, class and history* (Fontana, London, 1980), p.203.

6. D. Armstrong, *The first 50 years: a history of nursing at Royal Prince Alfred Hospital, Sydney from 1882–1932* (Royal Prince Alfred Hospital, Sydney, 1965).

7. The Wollongong Hospital, *Annual Reports* (1919–1952).

8. See Armstrong, *The first 50 years* and J. Castle, *Nursing at the Wollongong Hospital 1926–1982* (University of Wollongong Press, Wollongong, NSW, 1985), Chapter 2.

9. *ANJ*, vol.xxiii, no.2 (February 1935), pp.37–9.

10. *ANJ*, vol.xlvi, no. 3 (March 1948).

11. For example, at a large country hospital, Wollongong, *Annual Report* (1951).

12. Wollongong 1951 but at Royal Prince Alfred, a large metropolitan hospital, it was 1935. *ANJ*, vol.xxxiii, no.2 (February 1935), pp.37–8

13. Castle, *Nursing at the Wollongong Hospital*, pp.18–19.

14. Ibid., p.52.

15. Kelly Report, New South Wales *Parliamentary Papers* (1943–4).

16. *ANJ*, vol.xlvi, no.3 (March 1948), p.48.

17. *ANJ*, vol.xlvii, no.5 (May 1949), p.98.

18. *Report of the committee to consider all aspects of nursing*, part 1 (September 1937), p.31.

19. Ibid., p.37.

20. Commonwealth of Australia, *Parliamentary Report*, no.320 (1978).

21. *ANJ*, vol.xliv (August 1946), p.135.

22. M. Bush, 'Nursing as a feminist issue', *The Lamp* (April 1981), pp.25–9 (an article by a nurse counsellor); of the many academic articles see, for example, E. Lewin, 'Feminist ideology and the meaning of work: the case of nursing', *Catalyst*, no.8 (Winter 1974), pp.78–103.

23. Gamarnikow, 'Sexual division of labour'.

24. J. and O. Banks, *Feminism and family planning in Victorian England* (Liverpool University Press, Liverpool, 1964).

25. For example, at Wollongong Hospital there were six cases in 1927 and nine in 1928. See *Annual Reports* for those years.

26. A. Game and R. Pringle (eds), *Gender at work* (Allen and Unwin, Sydney, 1983), Chapter 5.

27. See Castle, *Nursing at the Wollongong Hospital*, Chapter 3.

28. See Castle, *Nursing at the Wollongong Hospital*, Chapter 3 and Game and Pringle, *Gender at work*, Chapter 4.

29. Castle, *Nursing at the Wollongong Hospital*, p.38.

30. *New South Wales Industrial Gazette* (October-December 1953), vol. III, p.218, clause 29.

31. Cited in Castle, *Nursing at Wollongong Hospital*, p.37.

32. Castle, *Nursing at the Wollongong Hospital*.

33. Ibid., p.51

34. Ibid., p.52.

35. Ibid., p.53.

36. Ibid., p.65.

37. Ibid., p.59.

38. Ibid., p.43.

39. Ibid., pp.42–3.

40. Ibid.

41. *Year Book of the Commonwealth of Australia (CYB)*, no. 33, no.40, p.700.

42. Ibid., p.46.

43. *New South Wales Year Book* (NSWYB), no.66 (1981), p.298 and *NSWYB*, no. 64 (1979), pp.517–18.

44. Ibid., p.705.

45. *Hospital nurses (state) award NSW* (1936), with amendments. All figures cited for nurses' pay and hours in 1936 are from this award.

46. *CYB*, p. 695.

47. Ibid., p.705.

48. Castle, *Nursing at the Wollongong Hospital*, p.46.

49. *ANJ*, vol.xxix, no.5 (May 1931).

50. 'A survey of Australian nursing education needs', *ANJ*, vol.xlvi, no.3 (March 1948), pp.48–51.

51. *ANJ*, vol.xxix, no.7 (July 1931), p.133.

52. Interview (March 1983), Mrs A. Jeffrey.

53. *Truth* (13 April 1927), the author was Mrs Jeffrey.

54. 'Origin of the NSW nurses association', *The Lamp* (May 1981), p.9.

55. Ibid.

56. Ibid.

57. *ANJ*, vol.xxix, no.7 (July 1931), p.133.

58. *The Lamp* (May 1981), p.10.

59. *ANJ*, vol.i, no.1 (March 1903), p.2.

60. *The Lamp* (May 1966), p.12.

3

The Nightingale Nurses:
The Myth and the Reality

Monica E. Baly

INTRODUCTION

The popular conception of the Nightingale reform of nursing is that it was planned by Miss Nightingale with her friend Mrs Wardroper and that it relied on supervision and elaborate character assessment. The idea that the school was revolutionary was implanted by Sir Edward Cook in his monumental biography of Florence Nightingale published in 1913 in which he says in an oft-quoted passage:

> Decidedly Miss Nightingale emphasised the educational side of her new experiment. No public school, university or other institution ever had so elaborate and exhaustive system of marks. Equally thorough and scientific are the General Directions which the Resident Medical Officer presently drew up at Miss Nightingale's earnest request.[1]

Sir Edward does not say, because he did not know, that Miss Nightingale complained that the assessment sheets 'were as capricious as if a cat had made them' and that the general directions drawn up by Mr Whitfield were quite unsuitable and that later 'he did nothing for the nurses'.[2]

In the preface to his two volumes, Sir Edward acknowledges his debt to Henry Bonham Carter, Miss Nightingale's cousin, her executor and the Secretary to the Nightingale Fund Council. The Nightingale archives are enormous and although the correspondence about the disputes over the training school exists, presumably Sir Edward did not see it. By now Henry Bonham Carter was over 80 years old and may have forgotten some things, he was a lawyer and would tread carefully and the relationship between the Fund and St Thomas's Hospital was in a delicate state.[3] More important, although the concept of nurse training had been accepted, it was still necessary to hammer home the message. Henry Bonham Carter had a vested interest in the 'steady progress towards the light' theory of history.

Nurse authors and historians at the beginning of the century had a similar interest; anxious to portray nursing as a homogeneous, educated profession they tended to exaggerate the revolution. Lavinia Dock, ignoring the fact that by 1900 the Nightingale School had only trained 982 nurses, wrote:

The master plan was brilliantly carried out . . . the whole existing system of nursing in civil hospitals was revolutionised by the introduction into them of trained, refined women. There was opposition at first but it gradually died away.[4]

Since then there have been over 20 full-length biographies of Miss Nightingale, but they have largely been a vision of Cook, and Mrs Woodham-Smith, as far as nursing is concerned, is no exception. Authors have either not read the archival material relating to nursing or have chosen to ignore it. In another context Lucy Seymer betrays that she has read the letters in which Miss Nightingale discusses Mr Whitfield's insobriety and that Mrs Wardroper was acting 'like an insane king' but she makes no reference to it.[5] This elliptical regard for historical accuracy, or carelessness, has done nursing a disservice. Instead of seeing the Nightingale reforms for what they were, a humble experiment, a compromise, and a battle between the Nightingale Fund and St Thomas's, the experiment was lauded into the 'Nightingale system' and ossified as tradition. Those who elevated the 1860 scheme into a blueprint for nurse training forgot that Miss Nightingale herself said 'we must proceed slowly and by experiment'.

THE NIGHTINGALE FUND

During the worst reverses of the Crimean War the grateful nation, under the guidance of Sidney Herbert, collected £45,000 for Miss Nightingale. The Council set up to administer the Fund decided that the money should be used 'to establish a permanent institution for the training, sustenance and protection of nurses and to arrange their proper employment'.[6] Miss Nightingale was contacted in Scutari about plans for the use of the Fund. She was not enthusiastic. 'Had I asked for money it would have been reasonable to ask for a prospectus of my plans', she replied and in a letter to Mrs Bracebridge she said:

If I had a plan it would simply be to take the poorest and least organised hospital in London and, putting myself there see what I could do, perhaps not touching the Fund for years till experience had shown how the Fund might best be available.[7]

Although suitably gracious in accepting the Fund, it is clear that Miss Nightingale feared it would divert her from her main purpose when she returned: the reform of the army medical services and, if necessary, the army itself.

Shortly after her return, while working on the Royal Commission, Miss Nightingale collapsed and took to her bed, and she then used her ill-health and the pressure of other work to do nothing about the Fund. She wrote to Sidney Herbert trying to divest herself of responsibility,[8] and even wrote her last will leaving the money to the Council. But Miss Nightingale did not die, and as she busied herself with other matters the Council began to consider ways of applying the money. One suggestion, dear to the High Church members of the Council, was that the Fund should be used to expand the work of the Sisters of St John who controlled the nursing at King's College Hospital.[9] Members of the Council made other suggestions but Miss Nightingale did not respond though she said she was applying to every hospital in London.

WHY ST THOMAS'S HOSPITAL?

At this stage Miss Nightingale was more interested in hospital building than in nursing and her advice was sought about the rebuilding of St Thomas's. Mr Whitfield, the resident medical officer, was interested in the idea of building hospitals on high healthy ground in the suburbs as proposed by Dr Farr and others, and he enlisted Miss Nightingale's support. Miss Nightingale saw the chance to 'build the finest hospital in Europe' on the pavilion lines of Lariboiseire away from the insanitary wen of London. The Nightingale-Whitfield proposals attracted a faction but this

35

was bitterly opposed by many of the medical staff at St Thomas's who insisted that St Thomas's must remain in the centre of London. During the course of the unedifying 'build in the suburbs' battle, there is a significant letter from Mr Whitfield to Miss Nightingale which suggests that he might persuade St Thomas's to accept a scheme for the use of the Fund. Miss Nightingale seems to have suggested her friend Dr Blackwell as the superintendent of nurses, but in a letter Mr Whitfield pointed out that she would be unacceptable to St Thomas's. Unfortunately we have not all Miss Nightingale's proposals, but she apparently sent him a scheme for training that he turned down.

> . . . the class of women who now supply the hospitals with sisters and nurses could or would not understand a hundreth part of what you wish to impress upon them . . . it would be impossible to find women capable of undertaking the competitive examination you have drawn out.[10]

After three years of inaction Miss Nightingale was being pressed by the Council to do something and she appears to have seen the St Thomas's offer as a way out of the dilemma. The Fund Council was not entirely happy, because part of the St Thomas's deal was that they must accept the matron, Mrs Wardroper, as head of the Council's school of nursing. Sir John McNeill wrote that she (Miss Nightingale) 'had a choice of beginning at St. Thomas's or waiting till you have trained some suitable matron' and he went on to imply that the second course might be better.[11]

But Miss Nightingale found the Fund a millstone that she wanted to offload and accepted it was 'not the best conceivable way of beginning, but the best possible'. Far from Miss Nightingale choosing St Thomas's because it was 'large, rich and well-managed' and because she admired Mrs Wardroper[12]; St Thomas's made an offer on *its* terms, one of which was that the 15 probationers under the Fund should be assistant nurses and have a contract to give service after they had finished training, and that the matron of the hospital must also be head of the training school. Once the preliminaries were agreed, Miss Nightingale wrote 'I must see the matron', which she did, and it seems discussed diets for nurses.

MISS NIGHTINGALE'S VIEWS ON NURSING IN 1860

Miss Nightingale had looked all over Europe and had had her own experience of nurses in the Crimea with the high attrition rate of nurses of all classes.[13] In her notes on *Different Systems of Nursing*, Miss Nightingale commended the system where 'Nurses belong to a religious organisation and are under their own spiritual head, the institution being administered by a separate, secular, governing body.'[14] and for this reason she was attracted to the system of St John's and King's College. But in the Crimea Miss Nightingale had seen what havoc lady ecclesiastics could wreak and she was determined that she must now avoid the *odium theologicum*; moreover, it is doubtful from subsequent evidence whether St John's would have accepted the conditions of the Nightingale Fund. What she wanted was the morality and spiritual devotion of religious orders, the education of the middle classes, combined with the hardiness of working-class girls. She knew from experience that such a synthesis would be difficult to find. By the time the contract with St Thomas's was drawn up Miss Nightingale, perhaps persuaded by Mr Whitfield, had come to the conclusion that working-class girls would be best for the experiment, and the original contract suggests that St Thomas's nurses might become Nightingale probationers. Miss Terrot was brought from King's College to help with the reading and writing. The probationers should work hard and set a moral example. In a letter to Mr Rathbone who was setting up a training school in Liverpool, she says:

A common day room is undesirable. It encourages dawdling and gossiping. Her (the nurse) time ought to be fully taken up with her ward work, her necessary sleep and exercise and what making and mending she has to do for herself . . .[15]

Hospitals were lawless, corrupting places and if nursing was to be reformed nurses must be kept away from corridors and stairs and from any chance of gossip or molestation, hence the need for a secure nurses' home.

The probationers selected by Mrs Wardroper had a harsh contract; they were paid £10 a year and a gratuity of £3 or £5 according to their class of award on evidence of their serving in a hospital for the poor sick following their training year. This gratuity helps the historian to trace what happened to the probationers after training (see Appendix). The Fund Council was paying the cost of the 15 assistant nurses in return for some not too clearly defined promise of instruction. St Thomas's had in the words of Sir Harry Verney later, 'driven a hard bargain'.

Not all the Council agreed with the contract. Mr Bracebridge protested about the autocratic power given to the matron, and Sir John McNeill demurred about the contract to give service as being unprofessional. All too soon, however, Miss Nightingale was to retreat into grief at the deaths of Sidney Herbert, the Chairman of the Fund, and Arthur Clough, her cousin by marriage and the first Secretary of the Fund. Having drawn up her famous assessment sheet with its 14 heads, Miss Nightingale was content to leave the school to Mrs Wardroper, Mr Bonham Carter, the new Secretary to the Fund and to visitations from various members of the Fund Council who were all eminent and busy people.

WHAT HAPPENED TO THE FIRST NIGHTINGALE NURSES?

Meanwhile, St Thomas's moved to Surrey Gardens and the probationers with it. From all accounts the conditions were difficult and often insanitary. Rachel Strong describes the 'balconies being used for sanitary purposes' and 'the ground floor where the ward kitchen was also the operating theatre'.[16] The Fund Council considered moving the school to Guy's Hospital but they had a contract with St Thomas's and there was the hope of the new hospital in the healthy suburbs — possibly Blackheath. Under these conditions it is small wonder that the probationers were often sick. In the first seven years there were fourteen diagnosed cases of typhoid, typhus, scarlet fever and diphtheria, with another sixteen off with fever. More than half the intake were off with sore throats, septic fingers and diarrhoea and some were off sick more than they were on duty. Elizabeth Pratt who contracted scarlet fever and diphtheria was dismissed for 'poor health' with the cryptic remark 'would have made a good nurse'. Of the first sixty probationers, three died. Nor does the recorded sickness tell the whole story because we know from probationers' letters that they treated one another.

Using the *Red Register* as a guide and excluding those who were dismissed before they could be recorded, there are 180 names for the first 10 years. Sixty-six did not complete their contract; four died in training; seven 'resigned' with no reason given. Of the others, half were dismissed for misconduct, with at least five for insobriety while the remainder were dismissed for poor health with some remark like 'not strong enough for our work'. The fact that so many were dismissed for glaring defects including phthisis, syphilis and drug addiction, seems to indicate that either Mrs Wardroper's judgement was poor; the references were dishonest; or there was no choice. Unfortunately, we do not know how many applications Mrs Wardroper received, but from Mr Bonham Carter's comments it would seem that the school attracted few suitable candidates.

THE FUND COUNCIL'S PUBLICITY

Nevertheless, in spite of the unspectacular beginning the Council members continued to claim that the scheme was revolutionary. They wrote letters to *The Times*, the medical journals, magazines and Sir Joshua Jebb, the Chairman of the Fund, addressed the prestigious Social Science Association, while Henry Bonham Carter produced pamphlets and authoritative articles. No breath of misgiving reached the public. Publicity brought a few better educated recruits, one was Agnes Jones, the niece of the Governor General of India, who had a religious call; some, like Florence Lees, came as observers and others by special arrangement, like Emma Rappe from Sweden and Jane Deeble from the War Office. With the exception of Agnes Jones, who Miss Nightingale feared having because of her preaching, they were critical of what they found. Miss Rappe wrote 'We did not learn this or that at St. Thomas's and there was not held a single lecture in anatomy or physiology while I was there.'[17] But Miss Rappe's and Mrs Deeble's complaints were dismissed because they were 'antagonistic to Mrs Wardroper'.

For a variety of reasons after 1867 Miss Nightingale gave more time to the school. For one thing, she was furious that the Governors decided to rebuild, not in the healthy suburbs, but on the banks of the dirty Thames, which she considered 'the worst site in London'[18], and she and her Council had to negotiate the building of special accommodation for the probationers.

St Thomas's, having realised the value of probationers, were now pressing for their number to be increased, but Miss Nightingale feared this because, as she commented more than once, 'the probationers were doing half the hospital's work'. Mr Bonham Carter pointed out that the Fund could only support ten probationers, but by now Miss Nightingale had come round to the view that the Fund should aim at better educated recruits in order to supply training sisters — 'we shall eventually come to paying for training', she wrote. Thus was born the idea of 'special probationers', paying for their board and lodging and, it was hoped, being groomed for superintendence. There was considerable criticism of the idea of ladies training with nurses but Miss Nightingale was adamant that 'the lady must be educated with her cook' and she would become a superintendent *because* she had done the same training and therefore know what was needed, and because she was educated. Educating the lady with her cook was to give rise to some problems especially when medical lectures became more esoteric, but Miss Nightingale did not change her view, thus giving nursing the tradition of a one portal of entry which lasted until the Nurses' Act of 1943.

Thanks to this publicity, the scheme attracted a few candidates though it must be admitted that their wastage rate was as high as that of the ordinary probationers. However, the new 'specials' saw Miss Nightingale and Mr Bonham Carter and they were articulate and critical. It was now clear that Mr Whitfield was not giving instruction as he was paid by the Fund to do, that practically no instruction was given on the wards and that 'Mrs Wardroper did not know one probationer from another'. It must, however, be remembered that Mrs Wardroper was not a nurse, did not pretend to be one and was the matron of a large hospital, responsible to the Treasurer for keeping down the costs.

The crisis came in 1871 when it was realised that the character and training assessment was quite unreliable and that Mr Whitfield did not fill in his space because he did not give lectures or know the probationers.[19] There was also criticism of Mrs Wardroper's relationship with Mr Whitfield which seemed to veer between being overclose and dominated by him, and jealous antagonism. Whether Mrs Wardroper was ill at this stage it is difficult to tell, she was certainly often off sick and Mr Bonham Carter seems to have taken over much of the decision making about probationers; he wrote 'I don't think Mrs Wardroper is able to form a sound judgement. I have not thought it prudent to discuss questions which require a good deal of calm consideration.'[20]

To overcome the difficulty, it was proposed to make Miss

Torrance, one of the specials, mistress of the probationers and to give them instruction both on the wards and in the home, but both Mrs Wardroper and Mr Whitfield forbade this and forbade her entrance to the hospital. In a long letter Miss Nightingale describes Mrs Wardroper as 'governing like a virago' and 'Mr Whitfield who has been for years in habits of intoxication. For years in the habit of making his rounds late at night, oftener tipsy than sober . . . at the same time his flirtations with Sister Butler were a current joke . . .'[21]

This was the end. Mr Bonham Carter asked for Mr Whitfield's resignation from the service of the Fund and after some unpleasantness, it was tendered. But what to do about Mrs Wardroper and the school? The Council considered moving elsewhere or spending all the capital and setting up an independent school, but Miss Nightingale was convinced that nursing could only be taught in a public hospital and who else would have them? Hospitals were not anxious to have a group of nurses not accountable to them. In the end there was a compromise and this is important because it produced much of what was regarded as the Nightingale tradition.

In order to keep the peace with Mrs Wardroper and the doctors, Miss Torrance became the home sister and was confined to giving lectures in the home and supervising nurses when off duty. Theoretical and practical instruction was divorced. Miss Nightingale protested but the Governors won. Miss Nightingale herself began to see the probationers regularly and started making her own comments in the *Red Register*, comments that often contradicted those of Mrs Wardroper. Mrs Wardroper was also summoned to South Street and from Miss Nightingale's notes we know that she was excitable, tearful and unable to express herself with brevity, but she was the matron of St Thomas's and she stayed until she retired at the age of 74 years in 1887.

Another measure to improve the standard of training was the appointment of Mr John Croft to give a course of instruction. Mr Croft's printed lectures are interesting because they indicate that the main admissions to St Thomas's were acute cases amenable to the surgery of the day. Although nursing points are emphasised, Mr Croft sees his brighter pupils as ancillary doctors able to take on the measuring and treatments previously done by doctors. The medical model had begun. Miss Nightingale herself was ambivalent; she once said:

experience teaches me that nursing and medicine must never be mixed up. It spoils both . . . I would say that the less knowledge of medicine a hospital matron has the better (1) because it does not improve her sanitary practice, (2) because it would make her miserable and intolerable to the doctors.[22]

On the other hand, she feared that if scientific lectures were not given, St Thomas's would fall behind other schools now being set up with ever more lady probationers who were capable of taking tasks from the doctors and anxious to do so.

So the Nightingale system evolved; everything was 'won at the point of a sword'. There was a secure nurses' home where a home sister looked after the moral welfare and gave some lectures, but who was divorced from the wards. Instruction on the wards was by ward sisters without any assurance that they had the ability, the time or the inclination to do so. Superintendents were raised to their position, not because they were specially prepared, but because they had a better education and background. Apart from a secure nurses' home, Miss Nightingale approved of none of these things, and there are pages of bitter correspondence about Miss Torrance's exclusion from teaching on the wards. In history, it often happens earlier than is thought. Contrary to popular belief, St Thomas's did not train to train. Miss Nightingale wrote 'I have said this scores of times, you must be tired of hearing me; *we do not* to those we expressly hold out a career of superintendence and training offer any special training'.[23]

From time to time the Fund tried to organise a course for superintendents but Mrs Wardroper always blocked the suggestion; the specials could not be spared from the wards. Those who came after showed no enthusiasm for special courses and towards the end of her life Miss Nightingale turned to other preoccupations.

Nevertheless, in spite of the lack of preparation the system did produce some pioneers, not because of what they learnt on the wards but because they were highly motivated, intelligent and had long talks with Miss Nightingale. Miss Pringle started a school in Edinburgh which was in some ways an advance on the school at St Thomas's with proper supervision at night and co-operation with colleges of education. Both Miss Torrance and Miss Vincent pioneered nurse training in Poor Law hospitals and laid the foundations for the nursing system in municipal hospitals. Nightingale nurses started schools in a variety of hospitals, though it must be confessed, some did not meet with Miss Nightingale's approval. But by the 1880s the gospel had spread and almost all teaching hospitals had lady probationers who went forth to pioneer nurse training, not alas, always as sanitary missioners to 'bring healthy habits and order to the lives of the poor' but to be acceptable assistants to doctors in hospitals now catering for the middle class. The biddable, young, neatly uniformed probationer was an asset to hospitals appealing for new clients. She was an even greater asset if she paid for her training.

However, the Nightingale system of sending out special probationers after a year in hospital as superintendents was not always the success that authors have made out. Miss Osburn, a cousin of Miss Nightingale, went out to Australia after eight months at St Thomas's and soon fell foul of the Fund by writing an indiscreet letter home about the attempted assassination of the Duke of Edinburgh who was nursed in her hospital. She stayed but was never forgiven. Miss Machin took a team to Canada but had endless disputes with the authorities and the experiment came to an untimely end. Miss Williams, Miss Nightingale's 'Goddess', had an unhappy spell as the matron of St Mary's in London where she clashed with the doctors and was forced to resign. Lucy Kidd was sent to replace the saintly Agnes Jones whose death left chaos, and was quickly dismissed for insobriety. Miss Barclay, a well-educated Quaker, was set to start a school in Edinburgh and within a year was forced to resign, a sad addict to opium and alcohol. The much admired Miss Torrance married and was in dispute with the Fund about her salary and Miss Nightingale never forgave her. And of Miss Merryweather, an observer, sent by Mr Rathbone to be the superintendent at Liverpool, Miss Nightingale was later to say 'does she know *anything* about nursing'.

The specials like the ordinary probationers worked as assistant nurses and were subject to the same, if not higher rate of iatric illness. A surprising number married which is not only a pointer to the late age of marriage in the later part of the nineteenth century, but also to the fact that life was not quite as vestal as the biographers made out, or as Mrs Wardroper tried to impose.

CONCLUSION

If we examine what the Nightingale School achieved in its early years, it is in fact very little. Most recruits were of much the same standard as nurses before the reforms, they did little formal training but they were subjected to greater discipline. Some had a vocation and learned what there was to learn and made good nurses. But after ten years Mr Bonham Carter was to write 'We have hitherto turned out only two good superintendents.'[24] One of these was Agnes Jones who, in spite of some success, was more concerned with 'bible work' and was unable to delegate.

Wherein, then, lay the success? The public relations machine is not new. While Miss Nightingale was complaining that Mrs Wardroper was behaving like 'a semi-insane king' and the Council was wondering if it could move the school elsewhere, the experiment was being trumpeted in the general press and the medical journals as a great success. In history what people think is happening is often as important as what actually happened. The Fund was inundated for advice from other hospitals, advice it freely gave, often putting up the standard of pay and accommodation offered to nurses and ensuring that they were always accountable to a trained nurse. This publicity, combined with the lack of opportunity for educated women made nursing 'fashionable' and attracted recruits not only to St Thomas's but to other teaching hospitals who saw the advantage of numbers of probationer nurses.

In some ways the Fund Council was caught in the web of its own cleverness. Having said the experiment was a success, they could hardly say that the system needed changing although at one point they considered spending capital and starting ' a school of our own'. What is interesting is that superintendents who came after Mrs Wardroper, and were trained nurses, saw no need to change the system. Obedience breeds an unquestioning conformity. Miss Nightingale wrote:

> If we had experienced sisters, if we had a matron with any system, if we had a Head to the Home, most certainly with 33–35 pros to 330 beds, at least 2 hours a day besides proper rest and exercises could be spared for each probationer for classes.[25]

But matrons at St Thomas's and elsewhere did not find two hours a day for classes nor did they allow a tutor on the wards; they were matrons of hospitals as well as heads of nurse training. Neither did they ensure that the ward sister set aside time for teaching; the diaries of specials in 1890 show that their day was almost entirely taken up with ward work. The needs of the hospital had triumphed.

By the 1890s Miss Nightingale had given up the unequal struggle and the Fund Council soon had to cede to less and less say as the hospital took on more and more probationers and the Fund could contribute to an even smaller proportion of their training. As Miss Nightingale said in a context elsewhere, 'sic transit *ingloria* mundi' (original emphasis).

The defects in nurse training highlighted in every report since the *Lancet* lie not in what was intended to be the 'Nightingale system' but in its abuse by the service needs of the hospital.

NOTES

1. Sir E. Cook, *The life of Florence Nightingale* (Macmillan, London, 1913), Vol.1, p.461.
2. F. Nightingale/H. Bonham Carter 18 May 1872. Greater London Record Office (GLRO). HI/ST/NC1. 72.12a
3. M. E. Baly, *Florence Nightingale and the nursing legacy* (Croom Helm, London, 1986), p.208f.
4. L. Dock and I. S. Stewart, *A short history of nursing*, 4th edn, (Putnam's Sons, London, 1920), p.126.
5. L. Seymer, *Florence Nightingale's nurses* (Pitman Press, London, 1960).
6. Nightingale Fund Council minutes. Resolution 8 November 1855.
7. F. Nightingale/S. Bracebridge February 1856. Sidney Herbert papers, Wilton House.
8. F. Nightingale/S. Herbert 23 March 1858. Sidney Herbert papers, Wilton House.
9. S. Herbert/F. Nightingale 22 March 1858. BL.Add.Mss. 43394 f21.
10. R. G. Whitfield/F. Nightingale 18 March 1859. BL.Add.Mss. 47742 f65.
11. Sir J. McNeill/F. Nightingale 11 April 1859. BL.Add.Mss. 45768 f94.
1. Cook, *Florence Nightingale*, Vol.1, p.458.
13. I. Palmer, *Florence Nightingale and the first organised delivery of nursing services* (AACN Publications, Washington, DC, 1983), pp.8–10.
14. F. Nightingale, *Notes on nursing* (1863 edn, Longman Green, London 1863), Appendix pp. 181–7.

15. F. Nightingale/W. Rathbone 20 June 1860. BL.Add.Mss. 47753 f1–7.

16. 'Recollections of Rachel Strong'. Unpublished typescript. GLRO HI/ST/NTS/Y/15

17. E. Rappe/F. Nightingale June 1867. BL.Add.Mss. 47759 f217.

18. F. Nightingale/R. Baggallay 13 January 1863. GLRO HI/ST/NCI/63.1.

19. F. Nightingale/H. Bonham Carter 24 November 1871. Bl.Add. Mss. 47716 f202.

20. F. Nightingale/H. Bonham Carter 2 February 1872. GLRO HI/ST/V 3/72.

21. F. Nightingale/H. Bonham Carter 18 May 1872. GLRO HI/ST/NCI/72 12a.

22. Z. Cope, *Florence Nightingale and the doctors* (Museum, London, 1954), p.121.

23. F. Nightingale/H. Bonham Carter 21 October 1876. BL.Add. Mss. 47719 f170.

24. H. Bonham Carter/W. Rathbone 1 October 1870. GLRO HI/ST/NC18 (11).

25. F. Nightingale/H. Bonham Carter 17 January 1873. BL.Add. Mss. 47717 f147.

26. Baly, *Florence Nightingale and the nursing legacy*, Appendix II, p. 232.

APPENDIX: What happened to the Nightingale nurses who entered training between 1860–7?

ENTERED TRAINING: JULY 1860 – JULY 1861

Reg. No.	Name	Age	Status	Health in Training	Training Report	Appointments (Contract) 1861-62	1862-63	1863-64	Subsequent Career
1	Mary Barker	32	S	Sore throat	Good	S.T.H. trans Netley.	Liverpool Work Ho.Inf.		1867 Sister Sydney Hosp. NSW; ret. Edinburgh in 1876
2	Jane Couchman	30	S	Sore throat	Good	S.T.H.(nurse) Liverpool Inf.		No further mention ?disappeared (no gratuity)	
3	Annie Lees	33	S	Sore throats	Good	S.T.H. trans Liverpool Work Ho.Inf. (left ill-health)		Rugby School (left ill-health)	
4	Emily Medhurst	25	S	Septic finger	Deficient in nicety	Bath (left - "no-one knows where")			
5	Maria Mullion	24	S	-	DISMISSED - DISOBEDIENCE				
6	Martha Murdoch	31	S	Pulmonary infection	DISMISSED - ILL HEALTH (?TB)				
7	Susan Newman	29	S	-	DISMISSED - INSOBRIETY				
8	Charlotte Nixon	31	S	-	Good - exceedingly good in all duties	Liverpool - DIED - TYPHUS (soon after arrival)			

Reg. No.	Name	Age	Status	Health in Training	Training Report	Appointments (Contract) 1861-62	1862-63	1863-64	Subsequent Career
9	Harriet Parker	25	S	Typhoid & scarlet fever	Generally good	Sick	S.T.H. – left the Service		
10	Mary Phillips	29	S	Jaundice bronchitis	Good	Warrington Work Ho. Inf. – ? (no further info.)			
11	Georgina Pike	29	S	Hysteria, sore throat	V.good – reported lectures well		S.T.H.	S.T.H.	?Left the Service
12	Elizabeth Stephens	29	S	RESIGNED					
13	Caroline Stone	22	S	Scalds, sore throat	V.good	Bath	Bath(Matron)	Bath(Matron)	Matron R.U.H. Bath
14	A.M. Tennant	40	W		DISMISSED – DISOBEDIENCE				
15	Emma Whitlock	34	S	Scarlet fever	Not strong enough, not educated	S.T.H. – LEFT – ILL-HEALTH			

ENTERED TRAINING: JULY 1861 – JANUARY 1862 (thereafter Register January to January)

Reg. No.	Name	Age	Status	Health in Training	Training Report	Appointments (Contract) 1862-63	1863-64	1864-65	Subsequent Career
16	Fanny Wilde	30	S	Sore throat	Good	S.T.H. – MARRIED			
17	Sarah Terrot	32	S	Sore throat, diarrhoea	Good	RESIGNED			
18	Elizabeth Perrottie	30	S	Sore throat, fever	Somewhat opinionated	S.T.H.	Leicester Infirmary (Head Nurse)	Devonport Hospital	
19	Ann Reilly	29	W		DISMISSED – INSOBRIETY				
20	Elizabeth Bane	40	W		RESIGNED – INCOMPETENT				

Reg. No.	Name	Age	Status	Health in Training	Training Report	Appointments (Contract) 1862-63	1863-64	1864-65	Subsequent Career
21	Mary Hind	34	W	Hepatitis, scarlet fever	Fairly good	Edinburgh Royal Infirmary	DISMISSED – FORGETFUL -------		
22	Helen Terrot	31	S	Returned to St John's House (special arrangement) to help with teaching spelling and reading				Came to St Thomas'	
23	Rebecca Riggott	32	S	Typhus, sore throat	Good		S.T.H./Nottingham/Woolwich Mil.Hosp.	Norwich Gen.Hosp.	
24	Margaret Garson	29	S	Typhus	Good	Liverpool W.H. Inf.	Devonport	?	
25	Elizabeth Cox	35	S	Bronchitis	Excellent	S.T.H.	S.T.H.	Addenbrookes (Sister)	
26	Deborah Burgess	34	S	Inflammation leg and foot	Good	S.T.H.	MARRIED -------		
27	Harriet Shooter	34	S		DISMISSED – INEFFICIENT				
28	Fanny Huston	35	S	Debility	Not strong enough	DIED – TYPHUS -------			
29	Jane Squires	37	S		Good	S.T.H. Dorset County MARRIED -------			
30	Annette Martin	29	S		Excellent	S.T.H.	S.T.H.	S.T.H.	Becomes Sister "Extra". Subject of FN's bitter attacks Left 1872
31	Anabelle Hickman		S		DISMISSED – UNSUITABLE -------				
32	Susan Hickman	31	S		DISMISSED – UNSUITABLE -------				

49

Reg. No.	Name	Age	Status	Health in Training	Training Report	Appointments (Contract) 1862-63	1863-64	1864-65	Subsequent Career
33	Ellen Powell	30	S.	Typhus	Good plain nurse	Liverpool Inf.	Liverpool	RESIGNED ------	
34	Elizabeth Wotton	26	S	Typhus	Good plain nurse	S.T.H.	S.T.H.	Addenbrookes (Sister)	
35	Elizabeth Kilovert	34	S		DISMISSED ------				

ENTERED TRAINING: JANUARY 1862 - 1863

Reg. No.	Name	Age	Status	Health in Training	Training Report	Appointments 1863	1864	1865	Subsequent Career
36	Henrietta Walker	34	S	Neuralgia, influenza	Good	Kings College	Liverpool Inf. (Nurse)		DIED 1921
37	Mary Merryweather	41	S	Only 2 months as a 'pupil' (sent by Mr Rathbone)			Lady Supt. Royal Inf. Liverpool		
38	Eliz. Merryweather	37	S	Only 2 months			Ass/Lady Supt. Royal Inf. Liverpool		
39	Emily Markham	23	S	Sore throat	Good, well informed	Cardiff Infirmary (Matron)			
40	Fanny Lovesay	33	W	Hepatitis debility	Good, superior education	Guys	Gen.Hospital, Salford (Matron)		
41	Mary Piety	33	S	Sore throat	F./good	DISMISSED - INDISCRETION OF CONDUCT TOWARDS STUDENTS ------			
42	Agnes Jones	29	S	Deafness, debility	Excellent	Supt., Northern Hospital	Lady Supt. Liverpool Work Ho. Inf.		DIED TYPHUS 1868
43	Betty Lillycrapp	33	S	Sore throat	Good	S.T.H.	Northampton Gen.		MARRIED
44	Helen Oliver	35	S			DISMISSED - IMPROPRIETY ?ALCOHOLISM, DRUG ADDICT ------			
45	Harriet Turner	23	S			DIED OF SCARLET FEVER - BURIED AT NORWOOD AT THE EXPENSE OF THE N.F.C. ------			

Reg. No.	Name	Age		Reason in Training	Training Report	1863	Appointments 1864	1865	Subsequent Career
46	Ann Batchford	31	S	Debility Chest infec.	DISMISSED – POOR HEALTH				
47	Caroline Blowman	24	S	?Phthisis	DISMISSED – POOR HEALTH				
48	Margaret Wilkes	29	W	Debility	DISMISSED – POOR HEALTH				

ENTERED TRAINING: JANUARY 1863 – 1864

Reg. No.	Name	Age		Reason in Training	Training Report	1864	Appointments 1865	1866	Subsequent Career
49	Anna Hearne	27	S	Billious	Satis. Poss. of making a good nurse	S.T.H. / Liverpool	Liverpool Work Ho.	County Hosp. Dorchester (Head Nurse)	
50	Fanny Beardmore	31	S		Good	S.T.H.	Liverpool Work Ho. Inf. (Head Nurse)	Liverpool	Not listed again
51					— MISSING —				
52	Nora Kennedy	27	S		DISMISSED – MORAL CHARACTER DEFECTIVE				
53	Mary Sales	37	S		DISMISSED – INSOBRIETY				
54	Hannah Frenfield	27	S		Very good	S.T.H.	Liverpool Work Ho. Inf. (Head Nurse)		
55	Mary Chalcroft	25	S	Colds	Satisfactory	S.T.H.	MARRIED		
56	Mary Chapman	27	S	Inflammation of the legs	Satisfactory	S.T.H.	MARRIED		
57	Mary Trueman	26	S	Headache	Satisfactory industrious	S.T.H.	Liverpool Work Ho. Inf.	Liverpool	Middlesex Hospital DISMISSED, UNFIT FOR SISTER'S POST

THE NIGHTINGALE NURSES

Reg. No.	Name	Age	Status	Health in Training	Training Report	1864	Appointments 1865	1866	Subsequent Career
58	Mary Snow	30	S		DIED OF TYPHOID				
59	Emma Flood	35	W	Colds	Good	S.T.H.	Liverpool Work Ho. Inf.	Liverpool	
60	Elizabeth Trueman	29	S		Good	S.T.H.	Liverpool Work Ho. Inf.	Liverpool	Middlesex Barts (Sister) DIED 1920
61	Elizabeth Harvey	27	S	Hysteria Haemorrhagia	Fair/good	Sick	S.T.H./Liverpool W.H.Inf.	Liverpool	Middlesex Hosp. DISMISSED – UNSUITABLE
62	Ann Tissington	24	S	Phthisis	DISMISSED – POOR HEALTH				
63	Maria Inwood	35	W	Typhus	Good	S.T.H.	Liverpool	DISMISSED	

ENTERED TRAINING: JANUARY 1864 – 1865

Reg. No.	Name	Age	Status	Health in Training	Training Report	1865	Appointments 1866	1867	Subsequent Career
64	Susan Jeans	24	S	Rheumatism Chest condition	Excellent	Liverpool Work Ho. Inf.			
65	Ann Burgess	32	W	Erysipilas and fever	Good	Liverpool Work Ho. Inf.	DISMISSED		
66	Ann Duffey	28	W	Colic	Good	S.T.H.	S.T.H.	S.T.H. MARRIED	
67	Emily Bull	29	S	Poisoned finger, fever	Good	Liverpool Work Ho. Inf.	Liverpool	S.T.H. (Sister)	
68	Emma Wilkington	41	Sep		DISMISSED AFTER A MONTH				
69	Angela Burcheur	36	Sep		DISMISSED				

Reg. No.	Name	Age	Status	Health in Training	Training Report	Appointments 1865	Appointments 1866	1867	Subsequent Career
70	Leonara Biscoe	39	S	Cold	Good	Addenbrookes DISMISSED	---		
71	Mary Silver	30	S	Sore throat Poisoned finger	Good	Stafford Inf.	Dorset County	Liverpool Hosp. Inf. Diseases (Matron)	
72	Lucy Emm	32	S	Cold Sore throat	Good	Liverpool Work Ho. Inf.	Liverpool Work Ho. Inf.	Netley (Head Nurse)	Left Netley 1876 - DISMISSED
73	Marion Bradbury	24	S		A fair nurse	S.T.H.	Cardiff Inf.	DIED ---	
74	Ann Blundell	27	W	Neuralgia	Moderate abilities	S.T.H.	Winchester	S.T.H. (Sister Adelaid)	
75	Louisa Francis	31	W	Billious	RESIGNED	---			
76	Sarah Dexter	29	S		Nervous temperament	Bradford (Matron)	RESIGNED - ILL HEALTH ---		
77	Elizabeth Foster	23	S	Sore throat	Moderate	S.T.H. (Nurse)	Manchester N. Assoc.		
78	Matilda West	27	S		A fair nurse	S.T.H.	Derby Inf. MARRIED ---		

ENTERED TRAINING: JANUARY 1865 - 1866

Reg. No.	Name	Age	Status	Health in Training	Training Report	Appointments 1866	Appointments 1867	1868	Subsequent Career
79	Anna Henna	32	S	Fever Sore throat	Good nurse	S.T.H.	Lincoln County DISMISSED ---		
80	S. Coulthord	29	S	Colic	Moderate	Manchester N. Assoc.			
81	Mary Wayte	30	S		Good	MARRIED ---			
82	Elizabeth Walton	30	S	Rheumatic fever	Good	Manchester N. Assoc. for Hospital Workers	Manchester		

Reg. No.	Name	Age	Status	Health in Training	Training Report	1866	Appointments 1867	1868	Subsequent Career
83	Sarah Henderson	33	S	Sore throat		Manchester N. Assoc.			
84	Mary Brieley	37	S	Erysipilas	Good	Manchester N. Assoc.			
85	Ellen Cullen	27	W	Colds/cough	Good	S.T.H. (Nurse) MARRIED ---------			
86	Agnes Lindsey	29	S	Accident Chest Inf.	F. good	S.T.H.	Margate Inf. Invalided		
87	Mary Rehnolds	24	S	Fever Sore throat	Moderate	S.T.H.	Winchester MARRIED --------- Inf.		
88	Emma Clark	24	S	Fever	Good plain nurse	S.T.H.	Derbyshire MARRIED County Hosp.		
89	Mary Mackie	33	S		Excited, nervous	Manchester N. Assoc.			
90	Ellen Rigley	34	S	Colds Billious	Good	S.T.H.	S.T.H./Swansea		
91	Alice Hubble	31	S		A plain nurse No particular ability	S.T.H.	Swansea (Head Nurse)		
92	Jane Bishop	21	S			S.T.H.	Winchester Inf. DISMISSED --------		
93	Elizabeth Blundell	26	W	Neuralgia	Plain nurse Good	S.T.H.	S.T.H. Sydney Hosp. DISMISSED -------- New South Wales		
94	Mary Farrell	20	S	Rheumatism	Moderate ability	S.T.H.	S.T.H./B.R.		
95	Ellen Dawtrey	33	W		Good	Margate Inf.	MARRIED ---------		

No.				Training	Report	1866	1867	1868	Subsequent Career
96	Betty Chaunt	28	W	Sore throat	Very good	S.T.H.	Derbyshire County	Sydney Hosp. New South Wales	DISMISSED --
97	Charlotte Wood	39	S	(Only 5 mths training)	Well educated Conscientious	Hampstead Union Superintendent	RESIGNED ---------		------
98	Elizabeth Goddard	33	W	Fever/cold	Ordinary capacity	S.T.H.			------
99	Mary Ward	33	S	Hepatitis	Intelligent Good nurse	S.T.H. (Sister)	DISMISSED FOR INSUBORDINATION, SOBRIETY DOUBTED ---------		------

ENTERED TRAINING: JANUARY 1866 - 1867

No.				Training	Report	Appointments 1867	1868	1869	Subsequent Career
100	Jane Markham	26	S	Neuralgia	Intelligent (Only 8 mths)	Swansea (Matron)			
101	Mary Gregory	26	W	Cold	Good plain nurse	S.T.H./ Derbyshire County Inf.	RESIGNED ---------		
102	Mary Barber	30	W	Colds	Good plain nurse	Lincoln County Inf.	RESIGNED ---------		
103	Annie Miller	32	S	Colds Sore throat	V.industrious Excellent surgical nurse	Derbyshire /Sydney Hospital County Inf./ New South Wales	DISMISSED ---------		
104	Annie Baster	34	S		Fair nurse	S.T.H. (Sister)			
105	Florence Lees	25	S		Well educated Fair surgical nurse	(Did very little training; did not comply with regulations)	S.T.H.		1874 Super/ Met.Nursing Assoc. Later - Mrs Darce Craven

Reg. No.	Name	Age	Status	Health in Training	Training Report	1867	Appointments 1868	1869	Subsequent Career
106	Elizabeth Young	31	W	Colds	Useful Intelligent	Netley/S.T.H. Devonport (Did part of training at Netley)			
107	Mary Bratstone	44	W		Good – part at Netley	Union Hampstead	Hampstead		
108	Mary Whitton	39	S	Operation for tumour	A person of mod.capacity	Lincoln/S.T.H. Blackburn (Matron)			
109	Emma Rapp	31	S		Well educated lady (8 mths only)	Returned to Sweden – Matron in Uppsala			
110	Elizabeth Kilvert	38	S	Cold/cough	5 mths train-ing only	Derbyshire County (Lady Superintendent)			
111	Helen Turriff	32	S	Cold	Good, intelligent	Sydney Hospital New South Wales (Sister) DISMISSED			
112	Mary Clark	35	S	Sore throat	Very good	S.T.H.	S.T.H.	Netley	
113	Mary Hart	34	S	Cold Sore throat	Plain nurse	S.T.H.	S.T.H.	S.T.H.	
114	Mary Butler	25	S	?Glandular fever/Irites	An intelligent nurse/good ability	S.T.H.	S.T.H.	S.T.H.	FN calls her 'an evil influence'
115	Lucy Osburn	29	S	Intermittent fever	Lady of sup-erior birth Mistress of several languages	Sydney Hospital, New South Wales (Lady Superintendent)			Stayed in NSW
116	Frances Smith	26	S		LEFT AFTER 4 MONTHS				
117	Clare Cullen	26	S	Sore throat	RESIGNED				

Reg. No.	Name	Age	Status	Health in Training	Training Report	1867	Appointments 1868	1869	Subsequent Career
118	Isabella Trydell	22	S	Cold	DISMISSED ON DISCLOSING SHE HAD ENGAGEMENT WITH ONE OF THE PORTERS ------				
119	Mary Reeves	25	S	Scarlet fever	Good	S.T.H.	Winchester County Hosp.		
120	Elizabeth Chung	25	S	Febricula	?	S.T.H.	Winchester County Hosp.	MARRIED ------	
121	Jane Williams	30	S		DISMISSED - UNSUITABLE ------				
122	Sarah Townsend	22	S	Scarlet fever	DISMISSED - NOT STRONG ENOUGH FOR THE WORK ------				
123	Charlotte Money	31	S	Infection of foot	DISMISSED - NOT STRONG ENOUGH FOR THE WORK ------				
124	Anna Reeves	33	W	Cold Sore throat	Plain nurse Moderate	Derby County			
125	C. Mottram	38	Sep		Incompetent	DISMISSED ------			
126	Ann Sullivan	38	W	Gastric derangement	Truthfulness doubtful	Blackburn (Head Nurse)			
127	Ann Nash	29	S	Cold	Moderate nurse	S.T.H.			
128	A.R. Jones	31	S	Debility	Good	?			

ENTERED TRAINING: JANUARY 1867 - 1868

Reg. No.	Name	Age	Status	Health in Training	Training Report		Appointments 1868	1869	1870
129	Lucy Kidd	31	S	Tonsillitis	Very good, exemplary character		1868	Liverpool (Lady Superintendent)	DISMISSED - MISCONDUCT ------
130	Lucy Stabler	30	W		Fairly good		S.T.H.	S.T.H.	

57

Reg. No.	Name	Age	Status	Health in Training	Training Report	Appointments 1868	1869	1870	Subsequent Career
131	Sarah Nash	32	S		DISMISSED - REFUSED TO SIGN AGREEMENT ----				
132	Mary Thomas	32	S	Sore throat	Fair ability Industrious	Gloucester Inf. (Superintendent)			
133	Harriet Elleman	41	S	Cold	RESIGNED - NOT STRONG ENOUGH ----				
134	Catherine Collins	29	W	Sore throat	Moderate abilities (mainly 'goods')	Derbyshire Inf. (Head Nurse)	DISMISSED - DISOBEDIENCE ----		
135	Rebecca Strong	23	M	Cold	Good practical nurse	Winchester	Netley	Netley	Matron, Glasgow Started 1st PTS 1880
136	Martha John	20	W	Febricula	?		S.T.H. MARRIED ----		
137	Julie Abbot	26	S		DIED OF TYPHOID				
138	Emma Berry	32	S	Cold	Fair nurse	S.T.H.	S.T.H.	Netley	Head Nurse Edinburgh 1876
139	Harriet Saunders	26	W		DISMISSED ----				
140	Jane Duke	37	S	Sore throat	Superior person	S.T.H. (Sister)	S.T.H. MARRIED ---- (Sister)		FN called her a bad influence
141	Margaret Westle	32	S	Cold	Good	S.T.H.	S.T.H.	Edinburgh	
142	Amelia Harris	42	S	Rheumatism	Plain nurse	S.T.H. RESIGNED ----			
143	Sarah Trueman	44	S	Fever	6 mth training	Matron at Winchester - special arrangement			

Reg. No.	Name	Age	Status	Health in Training	Training Report	1868	Appointments 1869	1870	Subsequent Career
144	Mary Winsall	35	S	Cold Sore throat	Fairly good	S.T.H.	Netley		
145	Sarah Litchfield	26	S	Febricula	RESIGNED – NOT STRONG ENOUGH FOR THE WORK ----------				
146	Henrietta Somerville	38	S		A lady of good ability	RESIGNED – NOT WILLING TO CONFORM WITH REGULATIONS ---------			
147	Catherine Tyrell	35	S	Colds	No comment	S.T.H.	ADMITTED AS A PATIENT TO BETHLEHEM ASYLUM ---		
148	Elizabeth Montforte	23	S	Colds	A woman of moderate ability	MARRIED -------------------------------------			

Source: M. E. Baly, 'A History of the Nightingale Fund Council, 1885–1914', unpublished thesis, (University of London), 1985. Appendix 9.

4

The Yale Experiment:
Innovation in Nursing Education

Sidney D. Krampitz

Florence Nightingale, in a 1893 letter to Tucker, a prominent leader in British nursing, writes '. . . It is for nurses to attend the outpatients and to teach the poor mothers how to manage their infants — how to feed, wash and clothe them . . . This is such a great item in the National Health and so neglected.' In America, during this same period, the establishment of sanatorium treatment for consumption and the adoption of the 'first comprehensive plan for dealing with the disease' made a significant contribution to the field of public health.[1]

The discovery of 'popular education' as an instrument in preventive medicine, made by those early pioneers in the tuberculosis movement, had proven that education was the *key* to a successful campaign to improve public health. Dr Hermann Biggs, a pioneer in public health in New York City, supported the appointment of school nurses in public schools in 1902, and a year later added public health nursing services to the 'municipal machinery for the control of tuberculosis', thus ushering in a new era for nursing practice and education.[2] Dr Winslow, in 1923, stated 'The public health nurse truly has become a central figure in the modern health campaign.'[3] He concurred with William Welch of Johns Hopkins, that America had 'made at least two unique contributions to the cause of public health — the Panama Canal and the public health nurse'.[4]

The growing awareness of the need for political and economic reform also provided additional pressure for change in the existing social system.[5] There was a general feeling of optimism that America could correct every social and economic injustice.[6] The impact of Progressivism and an increased awareness of the need for political and economic reform was to have an impact on

60

legislation which would significantly affect health care in America. The passage of the Sheppard-Towner Act provided for a rapid expansion of health conferences, development of centres for prenatal care and increased the scope of visiting nurse services.[7] This legislation, aimed at providing better health care for all Americans, necessitated immediate expansion and change in the existing system of nurse education.

As part of their general concern for the poor, reformers quickly recognised the contribution health education and nursing care could make in improving the living standards of the less fortunate. Society viewed professionals as altruists and experts and, therefore, looked to the professionals for leadership in dealing with its problems.[8] Social workers, having been actively involved in investigating the problems of the new immigrants and of the poor, recognised the need to send nurses into homes to provide direct nursing services for these families.

Nurses and physicians who were engaged in public health practice noted that adequate preparation for public health nursing could be obtained only by extensive revision of the nursing curriculum to include instruction in preventive medicine.[9] Although nurse education had moved in the 1870s from an apprenticeship style of education to training of nurses in a hospital school, the education of the nurse continued to focus almost exclusively on the care of acutely ill patients in hospitals. When nurses who had received such parochial training were faced with complex social, cultural, economic and environmental factors, they were poorly prepared to give the counselling and care required for preventive as well as curative practice. The collegiate schools of nursing had, from their inception, emphasised prevention of disability and disease; however, these fledgling schools had to augment their existing programmes in order to produce an adequate number of well-qualified nurse graduates to meet the changing and expanding needs for health care.

The rapid development of science and technology within the entire field of medicine made the revision and expansion of the nursing curriculum doubly imperative.[10] University affiliation for professional education became essential as professional practice increasingly demanded close relationships between applied or clinical practice and the basic scientific research which was becoming institutionalised in the American university.[11]

As the role of the nurse expanded, leaders in medicine also

recognised the need for broader educational preparation for nurses. Dr C-E. A. Winslow, a prominent leader in the American public health movement, addressing a professional group at the Pan-American Scientific Congress, stated:

> It is quite clear that the woman who enters the field of health nursing today is called to perform duties of a diverse sort, differing in marked degree from those performed by the bedside nurse of the past generation — to such a degree indeed almost to constitute this a new profession.[13]

William Welch identified the public health nurse as 'one of the very greatest agents in the advancement of health — both individual and public in America' and he strongly urged that the education of the nurse become an object of philanthropic support.[14]

THE ROCKEFELLER STUDY OF NURSING AND NURSING EDUCATION

The demand for public health nurses grew as the essential role they had in the rapidly growing public health movement became more apparent. Community leaders became increasingly concerned, not only regarding the services nurses could provide for the control and the prevention of disease in the homes of the poor, but also in providing protection from disease in all segments of the population. This growing interest in health education and preventive medicine placed ever greater responsibilities on the small number of nurses prepared for community practice.[15] Following the Conference on Public Health Nursing in 1918, the President of the Rockefeller Foundation appointed a committee to seek answers to the questions raised by the conference participants. This committee met in March 1919, and was formally recognised as the Committee for the Study of Public Health Nursing Education and subsequently funded by the Rockefeller Foundation. The initial committee consisted of leaders in nursing and medicine who strongly supported the university preparation for nursing.[16] The Committee, shortly after its establishment, was directed to expand the scope of the study to encompass a survey of the 'entire subject of nursing education'.[17] In June 1919, Josephine Goldman, a well-recognised social science researcher, assumed primary responsibility for organising and conducting this investigation of nursing and nursing education.

During this same period, a committee appointed by the American Medical Association (AMA) was also conducting a study of nursing. The American Medical Association's Committee on Trained Nursing was engaged in its study in the first year of the Rockefeller study and, in making its analysis, used materials made available by Goldman and the Committee on Nursing Education.[18] It is not surprising, therefore, to note many similarities in the findings of both groups. Both committees found major defects in the existing hospital training schools.[19]

At the annual meeting of the AMA in 1923, the Committee on Trained Nursing recommended that a minimum standard curriculum be established, that a means of enforcing standards be developed and that schools of nursing be established in colleges and universities to educate more and better prepared nursing faculty for existing hospital training schools. They further noted that basic nursing education in the hospital training school did not prepare nurses adequately for the increasing specialisation in nursing, and recommended that advanced courses be offered in 'special hospitals, in the hospital from which they graduated, or in the university schools of nursing'.[20] Thus, the AMA Committee did not recommend a major reform in the existing system of hospital training schools, but rather urged university preparation *only* for those nurses needing additional skills to assume management or teaching functions in specialised areas of nursing practice.

The Rockefeller study published its final report also in 1923, following several lengthy delays.[21] However, unlike the AMA study, the Rockefeller report identified the need for broad reform in nursing and nursing education. The study recognised the shortage of prepared nurses in the speciality of public health nursing as the 'largest outstanding problem before the health administrators of the present day' and recommended that all agencies employing public health nurses require not only a basic nursing education but also postgraduate instruction in public health nursing.[22] The failure to attract well-qualified students into the hospital training schools was seen as one outcome of an outdated apprenticeship style of education. In conclusion of their discussion of hospital training schools, the Study of Nursing and Nursing Education Committee stated that:

The average hospital training school is not organised on such a basis as to conform to standards accepted in other educational fields; that the instruction in such schools is frequently casual and uncorrelated; that the educational needs and the health and strength of students are frequently sacrificed to practical hospital exigencies; that such shortcomings are primarily due to lack of independent endowments for nursing education; that the existing educational facilities are on the whole in the majority of schools inadequate for the preparation . . . required for the care of serious illness and for service in the fields of public health nursing and nursing education.[23]

The findings of the study documented the unique advantages of a school of nursing established as an integral part of a college or university. Although the Study of Nursing Education did not recommend that all hospital training schools should establish courses of a character that a university would accept for a degree, it did identify the university school of nursing as the keystone of nursing education — not only training leaders in nursing but also greatly influencing the development of higher standards in all of nursing education. The Study of Nursing Education also emphasised the potential the university school of nursing had to 'influence' all of nursing education in America, and identified the need for an adequate endowment to develop undergraduate nursing programmes in universities.[24]

The expansion of nursing education in American colleges and universities was one outcome of this Study. This expansion was greatly facilitated by the growing interest of private philanthropy in nursing education. The establishment of undergraduate nursing programmes in two American universities immediately followed the publication of the Study. This paper will look at the establishment of nursing education at Yale University. That development was to have a major impact not only on the nursing profession but also on American higher education in general and was designed to become a 'model' programme of undergraduate nursing curriculum. The innovative methods used in the Yale programme gained wide acclaim. To understand this development at Yale in the 1920s, it becomes important to review also the status of medical education at Yale during this critical period and its relationship to nursing education.

In 1914, Dr George Blumer, Dean of the Yale Medical School, had recognised the opportunity public health nurses had to serve community needs and indicated this in a report to the President of Yale.[25] Several years later, Dan Blumer discussed the changes occurring in nursing education and stated that:

> the ideal situation in New Haven would be for the University to obtain sufficient endowment to put into operation a training school for nurses . . . which would rank as any other Department of the University and which would be on exactly the same basis as the other professional schools of the University.[26]

The following year the Annual Report of the Medical School indicated that a closer affiliation between the Yale Medical School and the Connecticut Training School for Nurses was being developed.[27] However, this affiliation did not change the focus of the hospital training programme and, therefore, failed to provide adequate training for public health nurses, a vision which had greatly influenced Dean Blumer's perspective.

In April 1918, a plan was formulated for the development of a university school of nursing at Yale. In this plan, the school of nursing was to have an affiliation with New Haven Hospital similar to the affiliation the hospital had with the Yale Medical School. This proposal was approved by a joint committee representing the Connecticut Training School, New Haven Hospital and Yale Medical School.[28] The rationale and plan for the establishment of nursing education at Yale was further developed and widely circulated in December 1918 to prominent public health nursing leaders and key professionals affiliated with existing university-based schools of nursing. This proposal contained several reasons why Yale University should proceed with the organisation of the school of nursing. The first was that the evolution of the medical school and hospital 'absolutely depends on the organisation of a strong school of nursing'.[29] The second reason identified was the need for academic reform in the apprenticeship system of nursing education. The proposal, therefore, recognised that nursing education was 'worthy of the highest tradition of public service of this University' and that Yale could take a leading position by initiating an experimental or model educational programme.[30] Shortly following the appointment of James Angell as the President of Yale University, Milton C. Winternitz, Dean of the Yale Medical School, considered the nursing situation at the New Haven Hospital critical and, in 1922, stated that 'the progress of the Medical School, particularly the clinical divisions, will be blocked unless there is a thorough reorganisation of the nursing situation'.[31]

Following the completion of the Rockefeller Study of Nursing and Nursing Education, a conference was held between Annie Goodrich, William Rappleye, Administrator of New Haven Hospital and Edwin R. Embree of the Rockefeller Foundation. At this conference a plan for the organisation of a collegiate nursing programme at Yale University was presented. Although Annie Goodrich indicated some reservations regarding the length of the proposed course, she expressed a willingness to undertake the experimental programme at Yale 'since greater opportunity for educational work would be available' and she regarded the experiment as 'the most significant of any which have been in nursing education'.[32]

Shortly after this conference, the Yale faculty submitted a formal proposal for the organisation of the Yale University School of Nursing.[33] This plan received wide support both within the university and from the Foundation. Abraham Flexner urged the support of the 'experimental demonstration' at Yale stating that the problems to be faced in New Haven 'are varied and representative, the Medical School group is a clear-headed, highly-trained, intelligent band, from which loyal, energetic, cooperative action is to be obtained'. He added that 'the President and Corporation are keenly interested in the Medical School and are giving time, thought, and money to it', thus implying this support would further aid Yale in the development of medical education.[34]

The Foundation directors had, in January 1922, 'approved in principle' a plan of 'cooperation in an experiment and demonstration in nurse training' which was to implement one of the major recommendations of the Rockefeller Study of Nursing and Nursing education.[35] At the annual meeting of the Foundation directors in 1923, after a review of proposals requesting Foundation support for the establishment of the reorganisation of various nursing programmes, the Rockefeller directors resolved to 'commit the Foundation to aid in the Experiment and Demonstration of Nurse Training under the auspices of Yale University over a period not to exceed five years and for a total sum not to exceed One Hundred Seventy-five Thousand Dollars ($175,000)'.[36] The initial Yale proposal included several features which the Foundation officers believed important in the reform of the existing apprenticeship system of nursing education. These features were:

> Emphasis upon education as contrasted with apprenticeship . . . Shortening of the time required for training, which would seem a natural corollary to increased educational opportunity . . . (and) Combination of instruction in bedside care and in public health service . . .[37]

Critical factors in the Foundation support of the Yale experiment were the appointment of Willard C. Rappleye as Superintendent of New Haven Hospital, the active interest of Dean Winternitz and President Angell of the University and, as stated by Hutchins in his *Report of the President of Yale*, the 'hearty willingness of the New Haven Visiting Nurses Association and the Connecticut Training School to throw their educational programmes into the hands of the new school . . .'[38]

The Yale Corporation, on 10 March 1923, voted to request the Rockefeller Foundation to contribute approximately $30,000 a year for not less than a five-year period for the establishment and maintenance of the educational proportion of a university school of nursing. The Rockefeller Foundation approved the request from the Yale Corporation. President Angell was then authorised to establish the Yale School of Nursing and to appoint a dean. Yale thus became one of the first undergraduate schools of nursing established as an integral part of an American university and its development had a major influence on the progress of nursing education in America.[39]

When the School of Nursing was established at Yale University in 1923, Annie Goodrich was appointed Dean of the School. Miss Goodrich was a widely-recognised nursing leader who had held several administrative positions in nursing and nursing education prior to her appointment at Yale.[40] Dean Goodrich had long been a strong proponent of university education for nursing and recognised the importance of the establishment of nursing programmes on an equal basis with other university professional schools.[41]

Upon accepting the appointment, Dean Goodrich immediately found herself in a situation in which the planned programme in nursing could not be carried out successfully with the funds available.[42] Although the Rockefeller Foundation had given a substantial annual appropriation to establish the School of Nursing at Yale University, unanticipated scholarship expenses and additional costs of faculty salaries and operating expenditures immcdiately created significant financial problems in the new programme.

However, the problem of obtaining adequate support for professional schools at Yale was not a new issue. Although the establishment of additional professional schools at Yale was 'clearly desirable', it was recognised that the existing endowments available to the university would not be adequate for unlimited expansion of these programmes.[43] An earlier president's *Report* (1914) outlined a policy for the development of professional schools in an endowed university. This report stated that the endowed university should give the professional schools:

> what they need to maintain the highest standard, but it should be understood that this aid is of a temporary nature . . . If after a certain length of time the work of any professional school does not appeal to the public, it seems inadmissable to make it a permanent burden upon other departments . . .[44]

Dr Farnam, Assistant Treasurer of the University, discussed the matter of endowment for the Yale School of Nursing and recommended a plan calling for two million dollars to enable long-term planning and development.[45] In 1929, the School of Nursing received a one million dollar endowment from the Rockefeller Foundation which assured its permanency at Yale University.[46]

Initially, the Yale experiment was filled with 'uncertainties' and 'was struggling against great odds' but, by the late 1920s, the school was widely acclaimed.[47] The Yale experiment was instrumental in initiating 'modifications in the nursing curriculum associated with outstanding nursing schools' throughout America.[48] The success of the Yale experiment resulted in the endowment of the School of Nursing by the Rockefeller Foundation.[49]

The support of the medical faculty at Yale for reform in nursing education is well documented. Milton Winternitz identified the relationship at Yale between the Dean of the School of Nursing and the Dean of the Medical School as 'the ideal' and stated that 'every effort is made to cooperate as far as the available personnel in one faculty might be of assistance in the teaching of the other'.[50] Upon Dean Goodrich's retirement,

Dean Winternitz remarked on the co-operation he had received from the School of Nursing and offered his continued support and assistance to the new Dean of Nursing at Yale.[51]

In 1934, college graduation became a prerequisite for admission to the Yale School of Nursing. This development again established a precedent in nursing education in America. Curti and Nash, in *Philanthropy in the Shaping of American Higher Education* (1965), identified the Yale plan of nursing education as 'revolutionary' and described this experiment as a:

demonstration that an educational experience free from control of hospital administration and medical staff would produce scientifically knowledgeable nurses who would carry on colleague relationships with other health professionals for the ultimate benefit of the general public.[52]

The Committee on Nursing Education of the American Medical Colleges made, in 1932, the following recommendations: 'the influence of the School of Medicine should increasingly pervade the development of the School of Nursing'; medical schools 'should use such additional university resources as may be necessary to bring their nursing schools up to the general level of the other colleges'; major emphasis should be placed on the development of 'adequate curriculum leading to the degree of Bachelor of Science, as well as other advanced curricula in various fields of specialised nursing endeavor'; and universities should 'accept the principle that courses in the curriculum of the School of Nursing be formulated and administered with the same seriousness and on the same collegiate levels as are demanded in accredited Colleges of Arts and Sciences . . .'[53]

The support of Drs Biggs, Winslow and others in the early days at Yale showed a commitment to a new vision of health care — that vision being preventive medicine. In his last public address, Dr Biggs again warned of the 'grave problems involved in the lack of sufficient numbers of well trained and qualified physicians and public health workers, and their proper distribution . . .'[54] The expansion of nursing and other support services again into patients homes during the 1980s due to DRGs and other economic and social pressures has broad implications for the education of the nurse practitioners of the future, and will again

69

challenge the nursing profession to seek now models for both undergraduate and graduate education in nursing.

NOTES

1. F. Nightingale/M. Tucker, 19 June 1893. Nightingale letters, History and Philosophy of Medicine Department, College of Health Sciences, University of Kansas, Kansas City, Kansas (NLK).
2. C-E. A. Winslow, *The evolution and significance of the modern public health campaign* (Yale University Press, New Haven, 1923), p.26.
3. C-E. A. Winslow, *The life of Hermann M. Biggs: physician and statesman of public health* (Lea and Febinger, Philadelphia, 1929), p.186.
4. Winslow, *The evolution and significance of the modern public health campaign*, p.56.
5. F. L. Allen, *Since yesterday: the 1930's in America* (Harper and Row, New York, 1939), p.89.
6. A. S. Link and W. P. Catton, *American epoch: a history of the United States since 1900*, 4th edn (Alfred A. Knopf, New York, 1973), p.3.
7. J. Stanley Lemons, *The woman citizen: social feminism in the 1920's* (University of Illinois Press, Chicago, 1973) pp.153–180.
8. Edgar H. Schein, *Professional education: some new directions* (McGraw-Hill Book Company, New York, 1972), p.2.
9. James E. Russell, 'The relationship of nursing to general education', *American Journal of Nursing* (10 July 1910), p.716; Louis Fitzpatrick, 'A history of the National Organisation for Public Health Nursing 1912–1952', dissertation, Teachers' College, Columbia University, 1972, p.413.
10. Lyndia Flanagan, *One strong voice: the story of the American nurses' association* (American Nurses' Association, Kansas City, Mo., 1976), p.21. Edgar Schein in *Professional Education* (1972) also recognises the growth and development of professions as a natural response to expanding knowledge and expressed societal needs.
11. Talcott Parsons and G.M. Platt, *The American University* (Harvard University Press, Cambridge, Mass., 1973), p.227.
12. M. A. Nutting, 'The social services of the district nurse', *Household Arts Review* (April 1910), p.8. See also Anne Bussell, 'The shortcomings of the teaching and methods of the present training-schools from the standpoint of the graduate nurse engaged in institutional work', *American Journal of Nursing* (4 January 1904), pp.267–70; Francis P. Denny, 'The need of an institution for the education of nurses independent of the hospitals', *Boston Medical and Surgical Journal*, 148 (January 1905), pp.657–9; E. McCraken, 'Public health nursing and the public', *The Modern Hospital* (9 October 1917), pp.297–9; M. A. Nutting, 'The training of nurses' in *A sound economic basis for schools of nursing and other addresses* (Putnam and Sons, New York, 1926),

pp.112–24; and Isabel Stewart, 'The educational value of the nurse in the public school' in *National society for the study of education, ninth year book, part II* (University of Chicago Press, Chicago, 1910), pp.58–9.

13. C-E. A. Winslow, 'The profession of public health nursing and its educational needs' in *Proceedings of the second Pan American Scientific Congress* (Government Printing Office, Washington, 1917), 5, pp.333–4.

14. W. H. Welch, 'Address to the graduating class, Johns Hopkins Hospital Training School for Nurses, May 1916', *The Johns Hopkins Nurses Alumnae Magazine* (15 August 1916), pp.144–5.

15. A. H. Strong, 'The nursing situation from the public health point of view, *Transactions of the American Hospital Association* (American Hospitals Association, Chicago, 1919), p.302.

16. Committee for the Study of Nursing Education, *Nursing and nursing education in the United States: report of the Committee for the Study of Nursing Education* (Macmillan, New York, 1923), p.1.

17. C-E. A. Winslow, 'Preliminary draft of report on the Committee for the Study of Nursing Education' (24 May 1922), p.2. Archives of the Department of Nursing Education, File 5, Drawer 2, Folder: Committee for the Study of Nursing Education, Teachers College, Columbia University, New York (Department of Nursing Archives). See also Rockefeller Foundation, Minutes of the Executive Committee, Meeting of 20 March 1919. Foundation Archives, 200 C Committee for the Study of Nursing Education 1918–19, RG 1.1, Series 200, Box 121, Folder 1494, Rockefeller Foundation Archives North Tarrytown, New York (Rockefeller Archives).

18. 'Preliminary report of the Committee on Trained Nursing to the Council of Medical Education and Hospitals of the American Medical Association', Department of Nursing Archives, 1922 (typescript), p.7, File 8, Drawer 2,. Folder: Report of AMA Committee on Trained Nursing (1922). Teachers College, Columbia University, New York.

19. Ibid., p.8.

20. Ibid., pp. 19–24.

21. Committee on the Study of Nursing Education, pp.97–106.

22. 'Report of Committee on Nursing Education' (22 June 1922), pp.2–3, Department of Nursing Archives, File 5, Drawer 1, Folder: Rockefeller Foundation, Conference and Plans. Teachers College, Columbia University, New York.

23. Ibid., p.12.

24. Ibid., pp.16–19.

25. *Report of the president of Yale University*, 11:221 (November 1914), Archives Sterling Library, Yale University, New Haven (Yale Archives).

26. *Report of the president of Yale University*, 13:292–3 (August 1917), Yale archives.

27. *Report of the president of Yale University*, 14:215 (August 1918), Yale Archives.

28. The plan, however, was found to pose some legal problems since the early charter of the Connecticut Training School and a subsequent

endowment by the school made it imperative that the training programme keep an independent board of trustees. For details of this early affiliation see the following: 'The proposal to make the school a department of the university', (typescript) (May 1918), Historical Collection, Box: Connecticut Training School for Nurses, Misc. 1873–1923, Folder: CIS and Plans for University Affiliation, Yale Medical Library, Yale University, New Haven: Leonard M. Daggett, 'Memorandum concerning proposed reorganisation of the Connecticut Training School for Nurses', (typescript) (11 May 1918), Yale Archives, Nursing Collection, Box 116, Folder 40.

29. 'An appeal for a university school of nursing' (typescript) (6 December 1918), p.6, Yale Archives, Nursing Collection, Box 116, Folder 40.

30. Ibid.

31. *Report of the president of Yale University*, 18:281 (September 1922), Yale Archives.

32. 'Conference concerning proposal for nurse training in New Haven' (1 February 1923). Rockefeller Archives, 200 C Yale University, 1920–1923. RG 1.1, Series 200, Box 123, Folder 1524.

33. 'Tentative outline of Yale University School of Nursing', (typescript) (12 February 1923), Yale Archives, Box 117, Folder 65.

34. 'Memorandum', Abraham Flexner to Edwin E. Embree (13 February 1923). Rockefeller Archives, 200 C Yale University School of Nursing 1920–1923. RG 1.1, Series 200, Box 123, Folder 1524.

35. The Rockefeller Foundation. Minutes of the Foundation, Meeting of 21 February 1923. Rockefeller Archives 200 C Yale University School of Nursing 1920–1923. RG 1.1, Series 200, Box 123, Folder 1524.

36. Ibid. See also the following letters located in the Rockefeller Archives, Nursing Collection, Box 117, Folder 65: Dr W. C. Rappleye, Yale Archives: Edwin E. Embree to W. C. Rappleye, 26 February 1923; W. C. Rappleye to A. Goodrich, 28 February 1923.

37. The Rockefeller Foundation. Minutes of 21 February 1923.

38. Dr Rappleye had previously been the Superintendent of the hospitals of the University of California and, while in that position, had actively engaged in a reorganisation of nurses' training to include community practice and social work. Rappleye had earlier conducted a study of hospital service and the training of hospital executives for the Rockefeller Foundation. See Edwin E. Embree/F. Elizabeth Crowell, 9 April 1923. Rockefeller Archives, Box 123, Folder 1524.

39. R. M. Hutchins, 'Report of the secretary', in *Report of the president of Yale University, 19:37 (September 1923), Yale Archives. See also Report of the president of Yale university*, 19:21 (September 1923), Yale Archives.

40. Following her graduation from New York Hospital in 1892, Miss Goodrich held the following positions: Superintendent of Nurses at New York Post-Graduate Hospital (1893–1900); Director of Henry Street Visiting Nurse Association (1917–23); Dean of the Army School of Nursing (1918–19); and the Lecturer and Professor of Nursing at Teachers' College, Columbia University, New York (1904–23). In

addition, she held the following elected positions in professional organisations: President, American Society of Superintendents of Training Schools for Nurses (1905–6); President, International Council of Nurses (1912–15); President, American Nurses Association (1916–18); and President, Association of Collegiate Schools of Nursing (1934–6).

41. Annie Goodrich, 'The university and the school of nursing', *Modern Hospital* (6 May 1916), p. 355.

42. Annie Goodrich/James Angell, 14 April 1924. Yale Archives, Box 117, Folder: James Angell 1923–34.

43. *Report of the President of Yale University*, 11:13 (November 1914), Yale Archives.

44. Ibid., p.15.

45. 'Endowment' (26 January 1927) (typescript) Yale Archives, Nursing Collection, Box 11, Folder: Endowment Fund 1926–27.

46. Brooks Mather Kelley, *Yale, a history* (Yale University Press, New Haven, 1974), p.383.

47. Effie Taylor, Nursing Director, New Haven Hospital/M. A.Nutting, 22 June 1923. Department of Nursing Archives, File 5, Drawer 1, Folder: National League of Nursing Education; Effie Taylor/ A. M. Nutting, 7 July 1924. Department of Nursing Archives, File 5, Drawer 1, Folder: National League of Nursing Education.

48. 'Dictated by Dan Winternitz' (9 April 1928) (typescript), Yale Archives, Nursing Collection, Box 117, Folder 56: Reports to the President.

49. M. C. Winternitz, Dean, Yale School of Medicine/Charles P. Emerson, Dean, Indiana School of Medicine (26 June 1929) Yale Archives, Nursing Collection, Box 10, Folder: Dean Winternitz.

50. The Rockefeller Foundation, Minutes of the Foundation, Meeting of 9 November 1928. Rockefeller Archives, 200 C Yale University School of Nursing 1920–1923. RG 1.1, Series 200, Box 200, Folder 1524.

51. M. C. Winternitz/Dean Taylor, 21 January 1935. Yale Archives, Nursing Collection, Box 10, Folder: Dean M. Winternitz.

52. Merle Curti and Roderick Nash, *Philanthropy in the shaping of American higher education* (Rutgers University Press, New Brunswick, NJ, 1965), p.109.

53. 'Report of the Committee on Nursing Education', *Journal of the Association of American Medical Colleges* (8 January 1933), pp. 37–8. See also E. P. Lyons, 'The concern of the medical school in nursing education', *Annual report 1933 and proceedings of the National League of Nursing Education, thirty-ninth convention* (The League, New York, 1933).

54. Winslow, *The life of Hermann M. Biggs*, p. 372.

5

Midwifery: Legal or Illegal?
A Case Study of an Accused, 1905

Alice Friedman

Since the beginning of the history of western mankind, democracies have based their governance upon the existence of legislative, executive and judicial elements of their countries. Normally, the legislature passes the laws, the executive carries them out and the judiciary rules on whether the individual law fits within the broad spectrum of the country's governance. Today's health policies result from those fundamental legal and political decisions. As our society experiences changes and new problems within the health care system arise to perplex us, interest is heightened in knowing what preceded these changes. The historical puzzle is particularly mystifying when an attempt is made to understand these policies and their origins.

Midwifery in the United States is an area of health policy determination that was an important feature of the social spectrum in the first decade of the twentieth century and continues into the eighth decade. The topic has been addressed in general terms by many scholars.[1] The specifics which address the process of change that midwifery experienced have not received the same amount of attention. This article is concerned with the case, *Commonwealth v. Porn*,[2] which set the tone for the contraction of midwifery in Massachusetts and many other states. The decision in that case marked the demise of midwifery in Massachusetts. The protagonist in the case was the Board of Registration in Medicine. The Board was the prosecutor of midwifery. The role of midwifery was taken by a player forgotten today, Hanna Porn.

Midwifery was never acknowledged by the social and political reformers in the United States as being worthy to have a distinct place in the health care system. Seldom is the topic, even today, indexed in either political, social or medical care texts in spite of its wide acceptance on the Continent. Reformers in the early part of the century attacked taxation inequalities and sought to regulate business and industrial monopolies. They established the first juvenile courts, set minimum standards for habitation and even abolished fireworks as maimers of children. None considered the real capacities of midwives or looked into the benefits of regulating midwifery. Rather than modernise the practice, Massachusetts embarked on a venture to eradicate it.

This is a case study of how one Massachusetts midwife was singled out, brought to criminal court and found guilty of the illegal practice of medicine. This case became a precedent for cases dealing with the charges of illegal practice of medicine for midwives, chiropractors, optometrists and others.[3] As recently as 1985, this case was cited in a court brief. In this case study, the defendant's history, the climate of medical practice in the early 1900s and the case itself will be presented. The historical information was assembled from summaries of court cases, newspaper articles, study of the social and political climate of Massachusetts and through personal interviews.

Immigrant groups swelled the number of midwives in Massachusetts at the beginning of the century. Daily, midwives presented an ever greater challenge to physicians who were striving for a larger practice for themselves and for the greater professionalisation of medicine. Midwives and physicians competed for the same clients. Families, particularly those new to America, continued to choose the midwife for attendance at childbirth. Tradition, a desire for a female attendant, less expensive care, familiarity with the neighbourhood midwife, were some of the reasons for this choice. Midwives were an economic challenge to physicians, not only because they charged less, but they limited the physician's access to the total family as future clients. Both midwives and physicians conducted the deliveries at home. The crucial issue between them was centred around who was to be the attendant. Accusations and perpetuation of the myth that midwives were inadequate practitioners did not influence the poor and the immigrant.

At this time, medical educators mostly from the Boston area where the prominent medical schools were established, recognised that steps had to be taken to eliminate the competition of non-doctor attendants at childbirth if they were to provide experiences for the doctor in training. A similar line of reasoning

75

was expressed by Dr Joseph Price in supporting the use of maternity hospitals for educational purposes. He said 'the rich have to take care of the poor, and I feel that the pauper element of society should be wisely and humanely used for educational purposes that we may have more finished doctors . . .'[4] The desperate need for clinical cases for students was also reflected in an arrangement by Dr David H. Storer, a chairman of the Obstetrics and Jurisprudence Department of Harvard Medical School, to pay practising physicians or the Boston Dispensary two dollars for every maternity case turned over to students.[5]

Many arguments were made in the United States about the future of the midwife. Kobrin identified that 'at one extreme were those who advocated outright abolition of midwives with legal prosecution of those who continue to practise. This was the official attitude in the state of Massachusetts . . .'[2] The legal prosecution of Hanna Porn, midwife, reflects this frame of mind.

Why it was Hanna Porn who was thrust into the notoriety is not definitely known. Speculations include the fact that she herself was seeking legal retribution from a physician for libel. Or was it because she had such a successful practice? It was rumoured that she made herself known when she sought legal opinion about her practice.[6] For whatever reason, her's became the test case in a state where there were at least a thousand other midwives. Unfortunately, Hanna Porn, like so many other women has left no written personal documents. From her actions, though, it can be deduced that she was a hard working woman, a fighter and proud of her work.

When Hanna Porn was brought to trial in 1905, she was 47 years old, had been married, but was living alone in Gardner, Massachusetts. She had emigrated from Finland in 1891 with her parents and a large, extended family. Many Finns had settled in Gardner,[8] a small industrial town in central Massachusetts. Many worked in the furniture factories and chair-making was a common occupation for the male wage earner. A weekly wage for industrial workers in that state in the 1900s was about nine dollars.[9]

At that time, there were no Finnish doctors, lawyers, or leading citizens in the town with the exception of the Minister of the Finnish Evangelical Church who was educated at the Chicago Theological Seminary. Hanna Porn also went to Chicago to complete a six months' course at the Midwife Institute in 1896.

In the year 1904, Hanna Porn delivered 65 babies.[10] This was about one-fifth of the total births in Gardner that year. In 66 per cent of the cases the parents of the newborn were from Finland, 15 per cent from Sweden and the others predominately from Russia, and were Jewish. The homes in which she delivered babies were clustered mainly in the neighbourhood where the Finnish population had settled. She also lived there in one of the tenements. It was not uncommon for her to have several confinements on one street in the same month. One year she attended nine deliveries on Pleasant Street and the next year there were seven on the same street. Many of her patients were related to each other. This suggests a good reputation among the childbearing population. Her nephew, interviewed in his ninety-eighth year, and remembering the Gardner of his boyhood, said she was very popular and families were always seeking her care. He didn't know 'why the doctors were angry with her.'[11]

At no time in any of the public documents was there any allegations that Hanna Porn's practice was anything but of the highest quality. The judge in writing his final opinion on the case in 1907, added 'whatever hardship there may be upon the defendant who is a woman of good character and reputation as shown by the agreed upon facts, comes (only) from the scope of the statute'.[12]

It was a surprise to the readers in Gardner in 1905 when the local newspaper on 2 August, headlined a first page article: MIDWIFE CHARGED WITH BREAKING THE LAW PEOPLE ASSUMED THAT SHE HAD A PERMIT FROM STATE BOARD.[13] The article stated that only one physician in Gardner had registered a larger number of births than Mrs Porn. The reporter commented:

it is thought that the local authorities and physicians exhibited an extremely lenient spirit by not moving the matter until requested to do so by the Board of Registration (in Medicine); providing the law had been so flagrantly violated, as alleged.[14]

Mrs Porn had never concealed her identity from those interested in local medical affairs. On the brass nameplate on her door was the lettering, 'Mrs Porn, Midwife'. Her name appeared frequently on town records. She, like others who registered births were reimbursed by the town for conforming with the state regulation of Chapter 444, Acts of 1897:

An Act Relative to the Registry and Return of Births, Marriages, and Deaths.
Sec 3. Physicians and Midwives shall on or before the 5th day of each month report to the Clerk of each town a correct list of all children born . . . and where they were present.

With such a regulation, the town officials assumed that it was proper for midwives to attend births. The annual town budget in Gardner reflected payment for those birth certificates that Mrs Porn had submitted.

The registration forms that Mrs Porn completed were all carefully done and were outstanding because of her very neat and legible script. These were promptly completed at the town hall. On the forms, after 1905, she began to cross out 'physician' and write 'midwife' in the proper place for the attendant's signature.

All the deliveries that Mrs Porn attended were home births. There was no hospital in Gardner until 1907. The two patients who had hospital deliveries in 1904 went to Worcester, a city about 25 miles distant.

There were 16 physicians in Gardner in 1904.[15] Nine were members of the Massachusetts Medical Society. The Society, like the American Medical Society, was willing to develop, in conjunction with the government, methods by which the practice of medicine would be protected in its professional and economic standards. On the other hand, the Association had strong feelings as to how this protection was to be exercised. It was concerned that governmental action should not interfere with the exercise of what the physicians perceived as their rights of practice. They favoured medical control of licensure.

Three months prior to Hanna Porn's arrest, one local physician was elected president of the county branch of this society. At the meeting when the election took place, a medical speaker from Boston addressed the Society on the topic of 'Medical Organisation'.[16] How to achieve greater self-regulation of private medicine and how to eliminate non-doctor competition interested such groups.

An important part of this study lies in the role of the Board of Registration in Medicine. This Board was created in 1894,[17] by an Act of the state legislature. An earlier Bill, introduced in 1885 by the Massachusetts Medical Society had met with opposition.[18] Nine years later the Society was ready to compromise on its demands, and joined by public health officials, proposed legislation to register certain persons as physicians. Registered physicians would be allowed to practise medicine and others would be denied the privilege. The justification was that a high standard of professional qualification for physicians was of vital concern to the public health and that physicians, selected by the executive branch of the government, were the best determiners of those qualifications. This Act, which created state regulations, significantly altered health practices in the Commonwealth from that time onward. Organised medicine also reaped rewards as it was given the power to determine the scope of the practice of medicine. The process of the professionalisation of medicine was hastened. The public received symbolic benefits, but those who initiated the legislation shared in much of the material benefits.

The original members of the Board of Registration in Medicine were appointed by Governor Frederick T. Greenhalge, a Republican lawyer from Lowell. All members were physicians and all were male. A compromise in membership was reached as three positions were allocated to the Massachusetts Medical Society, two to the Massachusetts Homeopathic Medical Society and two to the Massachusetts Eclectic Society. Allopathic (or regular) physicians representing the Massachusetts Medical Society eventually became the sole members of the Board.

The Board had the discretionary power to issue registrations to those whom members agreed should practise medicine in Massachusetts. The Board defined medicine as 'the science which relates to the prevention, cure, or alleviation of disease'. Exempted from the law were clairvoyants, hypnotists, magnetic healers, mind curers, masseurs, Christian Scientists and cosmopathics. *Commonwealth v. Porn* became the classic case in which midwifery was declared not exempted from the law.

Three classes of registration were provided for those who could prove that they had been practising medicine for three years (the 'grandfathering' clause), for those graduates of legally chartered medical colleges or universities having the power to confer degrees in medicine and for those not included in the former classes but who passed an examination by the Board. Some who received a licence to practise were not graduates of medical schools, few of them had any college education and high school education was only 'recommended' as a prerequisite. Proof of a command of the English language was added later. Individuals who were so licensed had the privilege of practising medicine in Massachusetts indefinitely.

The medical leaders recognised that without a requirement of medical school graduation for physician registration, Massachusetts was classed in the company of such states as Arkansas, Mississippi and Tennessee in its backwardness. Massachusetts was still loitering in the background of progress in the medical world but attempts to pass stiffer requirements were abandoned. The withdrawal of such a proposal from the legislative docket suggests that the Board was doubtful of its success in upgrading practice through the legislature.

The political climate of the state at this time is described by Richard Abrams,[19] the historian, in his claim that 'Massachusetts never caught the spirit of change which dominated the era, and consequently appeared, at best, merely conservative.' Values which led to the acceptance of greater controls such as reliance upon qualified experts, for example the physicians as exclusive members of the Board; the wish to leave policy matters to the scientific community; the feeling that only the experts could master information too complicated for the lay person, were certainly in the conservative vein and made the government in many instances more responsive to the educated than to the democratic majority. There was faith in the elite and the medical elite was anxious to assume the leadership in health care decisions.

At this time the public health officials supported state regulation for sanitation, pure water, proper sewage disposal but not for state decisions regarding medical practices.[20] Midwives and nurses were not licensed, although nurses first attempted such legislation in 1902 and were opposed by the physicians.

The Board of Health did not seem to play an active part in examining the multiple causes of the high maternal mortality rate in Massachusetts. Not many years later, in New Jersey,[21] the public health officials through studies found that their midwives had better rates than did physicians in the case of maternal infections. Massachusetts allowed the myth to be perpetuated that such faults lay at the doorstep of the midwives. Physicians in Massachusetts complimented themselves on 'keeping politics out of (Massachusetts) public health'. The absence of political controversy was not surprising considering the mutuality of interests of the medical community with the Republican party in control of the State government.

The Chairman of the State Board of Health at this time was

Henry P. Walcott,[22] a physician. He was also Overseer of Harvard University, a fellow of the Harvard University Corporation and the liaison with President Eliot of Harvard relative to the Medical School. He was keenly aware of the efforts to raise the standards of Harvard Medical School. A revamped medical practice in the state was a prime consideration. A properly constituted Board of Medicine with members favouring this approach was the first step. Another was to eliminate the non-physician providers. The formidable task that Massachusetts was facing at this time was to improve the quality of physician. Outlawing the non-doctor attendant for instance in the field of obstetrics/midwifery without graduating and licensing well-qualified physicians was of limited effectiveness. Obstetrical education had to be improved. President Eliot in wielding a 'new broom'[23] at Harvard Medical School held the opinion that 'the medical students were noticeably inferior in bearing, manners and discipline'. He judged the average graduate of an American medical school to be ignorant and generally unskillful. He believed that the incompetence of the graduate when he receives his degree which 'turns him loose upon the community is something horrible to contemplate. The mistakes of an ignorant or stupid young physician or surgeon mean poisoning, maiming, or killing.'

A few years later, Abraham Flexner in his famous exposé of medical schools,[24] commented that the obstetrical training that most medical students received were the worst in their curriculum. In his memoirs, a physician recalls these inadequacies. Typically, the student in the obstetrics course in Boston would first have a few lectures on the theory of obstetrics and a demonstration of the birth process by use of a doll being passed through the broken crown of a straw hat. In addition, the student had four hours of clinical instruction at a hospital and then ten days direct experience with delivering babies in their own homes while he served as an externe. If he was lucky, he watched another externe deliver a baby before he was called upon to do so.

As an externe, attending the birth of babies in their homes was frequently his first experience with extreme poverty. These brief days 'on the district' showed him the horrible living conditions of the poor and immigrant. It was probably also upsetting to the student to recall his instructor's dictum for the 'absolute necessity for maintaining surgical cleanliness' as he was confronted with the horrid environment in the typical tenement.

Lack of knowledge of the social conditions of the poor was a definite handicap. The medical student experiencing his first delivery situation, was also undergoing his first intimate contact with people of different economic and social classes, with those of different cultures and with those of differing religious beliefs. Lack of knowledge of how immigrants lived sometimes bred lack of sympathy and tolerance. Compared with the familiar midwife who shared the cultural background and who could speak the native languages, it is understandable that given a choice, the poor and the immigrant chose the midwife.

The student's middle-class anti-immigrant prejudices also went with him as he visited his patients in labour. Recalling his externe day, one writer[25] said 'the Immigration Exclusion Act of 1921 was one of the few real statesman like acts on the part of Congress'. He also spoke of the Russian Jews and the Irish as the most dirty, the Sicilians as excitable and the Poles and Lithuanians as a group who were stupid, stubborn, difficult to handle and most likely to resort to violence, as he remembered his patients and their families.

Those wishing to replace the midwife at this time with a scientifically trained doctor acted with arrogance, power and haste. In spite of intentions, the evidence points to inadequately prepared persons being licensed as physicians. Even the physicians with the 'best' training in obstetrics were found lacking in their scientific preparation. The haste to drive the non-doctor practitioner from the field, motivated the outlawing of midwifery before another system to care for mothers and babies was in place.

The court action in the case *Commonwealth v. Porn* was initiated by the Board of Registration in Medicine. The Board, as part of the regulatory responsibilities of the executive branch of government, was located in Boston. The Board, after the alleged violation of Hanna Porn was brought to its attention, reported this to the authorities in Gardner, Massachusetts where Mrs Porn resided. A constable served notice on her. The case was heard in District Court, Gardner County Courthouse. The defence attorney tried to show through expert witnesses, two physicians, that the practice of midwifery was not the practice of medicine and therefore midwifery was not a violation of the medical registration act. The district attorney argued that whether the practice of midwifery was the practice of medicine was a question of law. Expert evidence was not admissable under those circumstances.

The judge upheld the district attorney, the expert witnesses were not allowed to testify. Mrs Porn was found guilty on 25 October 1905 and was fined one hundred dollars. The judge ruled that the practice of midwifery *was* the practice of medicine.

The decision was appealed. One and a half years later, in the Supreme Judicial Court in Worcester, the judge agreed with Mrs Porn's lawyer that the expert evidence should have been accepted. The purpose of that evidence would have been to show 'what a midwife does or is expected to do as such, so that the court may see whether her acts or any of them are to be regarded as the practice of medicine in any of its branches'. The conviction of 1905 was set aside.[26]

Another trial was held on 3 June 1907 in the Superior Court in Worcester. At that trial, Porn's lawyer was able to present a statement of facts to the judge and jury. On the basis of these facts, Judge John A. Aiken directed the jury to find the defendant guilty. The facts presented in Hanna Porn's defence were as follows:

1. She was a trained nurse.
2. She was a graduate of the Chicago Midwife Institute and therefore a graduate midwife who had received six months theoretical and practical instruction in the art of midwifery.
3. She delivered women for compensation.
4. She did not claim to be a general practitioner of medicine.
5. She carried with her the usual obstetrical instruments but she used these but rarely on occasions of emergency but never if a physician could be called.
6. She used six printed prescriptions of formulas for treating vaginal douche, postpartum haemorrhage, to prevent purulent ophthalmia in the newborn, for 'after pains', for uterine inertia, for painful haemorrhoids.

The defence attorney offered to show by expert witness that Mrs Porn did not hold herself out as a practitioner of medicine. The defence was refused, the judge referred to a case in 1835 when Chief Justice Leonard Shaw found that it was not necessary to 'profess' to practise generally to be considered under the regulatory statute. The jury found the defendant guilty and the decision was again appealed.

The Supreme Judicial Court, speaking through Justice Arthur Rugg, handed down its decision on 15 October 1907. The judge interpreted that Hanna Porn had indeed been engaged in the illegal practice of medicine as defined by the Statute of 1894. The judge pointed out that the facts in the case were undisputed, and he decided that the facts pointed to a violation of the Statute. Statements in support of this finding include the following: 'Both medical and popular lexicographics define midwife as a female obstetrician and midwifery as the practice of obstetrics' and 'Although childbirth is not a disease, but a normal function of women — obstetrics as a matter of common knowledge has long been treated as a highly important branch of the science of medicine.' Midwifery under this interpretation was the practice of medicine. Hanna Porn, having engaged in midwifery, was in fact practising medicine without a licence.

Porn's lawyer also contended that the Statute regulating the practice of medicine was unconstitutional. He was asking if legislating the exclusive right to practise 'the science which relates to the prevention, cure, or alleviation of disease' to physicians was in accordance with the constitution of the United States? Could it be interpreted as restraining business practices like a monopoly? The court overruled his contention and found that the state was protecting the public with its reasonable regulations for licensing physicians and to this end did not contravene any provision of the state or Federal constitution. The objection was overruled and the guilty verdict was left standing.

Midwifery was outlawed in Massachusetts but it continued to be practised here many years after the court decision. To implement the decision on a state-wide basis would have required additional resources. Not only were alternative services for maternity care not available, but local officials did not have the money nor manpower to enforce criminal actions against the many still practising midwives. In 1912, for instance of a total of 14,336 births in the combined cities of Fall River, New Bedford, Lawrence and Lowell, 24 per cent or more than 3000 births were attended by midwives. Local officials were reluctant to take adversary stand against the popular wishes of their constituents.

The law did slow down the growth of midwifery, for no professional midwife would set up practice in a state under this law. With a decrease in immigration and thus fewer additional midwives coming with these groups, attrition of their numbers took place. No Statute to license midwives was enacted. The Justice giving his decision in 1907 pointed out that the Legislature could create such a board which would make midwifery legal by statutory demarcation from the practice of medicine.

Opposing such legislation was a leading Boston obstetrician, James Huntington,[27] who frequently spoke out to women's groups in opposition to such licensing. Worcester, a leading physician from eastern Massachusetts, wanted the midwife to disappear and in her place develop a role of 'obstetric nurses'. Such a person would care for the woman in labour and then call in the physician for the delivery. He was looking for an assistant and was opposed to the autonomous role of the midwife.

The significance of the case, *Commonwealth v. Porn*, was the judicial finding that midwifery was the practice of medicine.

Many hold that the justice's finding was wrong, that midwifery, historically preceded obstetrics and therefore could not be part of its totality. The finding still holds, minimally it did serve to achieve a sense of order in the turbulent health care field of the 1900s. It did establish order but at the expense of the individual's choice of childbirth attendant. One hundred years later, the health care field reflects the narrowness of the scope of medicine which the decision in *Commonwealth v. Porn* guaranteed.

In the *Commonwealth v. Porn* case, the white, male, educated, socially-connected, mainly Boston elite of the medical profession, striving to raise the standards of obstetrics and medical education acted to abolish midwifery in Massachusetts through the application of the law. Through this strategy, midwifery was declared a crime and its decline in Massachusetts became a certainty. The decline was not immediate. Many women in childbirth continued to choose the midwife as their attendant. A reasonable compromise of educating and regulating the midwife's practice was opposed by the powerful medical leadership. Lacking the force of its own organisation of midwives; of a women's movement for support; and without a united voice for either the consumer or the foreign-born, 'stamping out midwifery' became a reality.

Hanna Porn believing that the law was unjust, continued to practise midwifery after 1907.[28] That year she delivered 70 babies. She was arrested again and this time was sentenced to three months in the House of Corrections. She died four years later, at the age of 53. Her death certificate listed her occupation as 'nurse'.

NOTES

1. Jane Pachet Brickman, 'Public health nurses, midwives and nurses, 1880–1930' in Ellen Condliffe Langemann (ed.), *Nursing history* (Teachers' College Press, New York, 1983), pp.65–88; Frances Kobrin, 'The American midwife controversy: a crisis of professionalization' in Judith W. Leavitt and Ronald Numbers (eds), *Sickness and health in America* (University of Wisconsin Press, Madison, Wisconsin, 1978), pp.217–25; R. W. Wertz and D. C. Wertz, *Lying-in: a history of childbirth in America* (Schoken Books, New York, 1979).

2. *Commonwealth v. Porn*, 195 Mass. 433 (1907).

3. *Crees v. California*, 28 Cal. Rptr 621; Lutheran Hospital etc., and Dept. of P. W. (Ind) 397, N E ed 638; *Banti v. State*, 289 S we 244.

4. Joseph Price, 'Obstetrical asepsis', *Boston Medical and Surgical Journal*, cxxxi, no.2 (11 January 1894), pp.40–2

5. Herbert Thoms, *Chapter in American obstetrics* (Thomas, Springfield, I., 1961), p.148.

6. *Gardner News* (21 June 1984).

7. Register of Death Certificates, Office of City Clerk, Gardner, Mass.

8. Doris Kirkpatrick, *Across the world in Fitchburg* (Fitchburg Historical Association, Fitchburg, 1975), Vol.II, pp.115–29.

9. *Thirty-Seventh Annual Report of the Bureau of the Statistics of Labor* (Wright and Potter, Boston, Mass., 1907), p.296.

10. Register of Birth Certificates, Office of the City Clerk, Gardner, Mass.

11. Personal interview with nephew (aged 98) of Hannah Porn, Eastwood Pines Nursing Home, Gardner, Mass.

12. *Commonwealth v. Porn*, 196 Mass. 326 (1907).

13. *Gardner News* (2 August 1905).

14. Ibid.

15. *Gardner Directory, 1905–1906* (New Haven, Conn., 1907), p.48.

16. *Gardner News* (25 April 1905).

17. Secretary of the Commonwealth, *Annual reports of the various public officers and institutions, 1894* (Boston, Mass., 1895), vol.iv, p.10.

18. *Boston Daily Globe* (8 June 1885). 'Remonstrant' wrote a letter to the newspaper beginning with 'I see the Massachusetts Medical Society after its long silent and desperate effort, has succeeded in inducing the committee (public health) to report a bill . . . an opening wedge as they call it. As one of the tens of thousands of remonstrants against this measure, I would appeal to the Legislature to act as the people wish, and not legislate for the doctors . . .'

19. Richard Abrams, *Conservatism in a progressive era: Massachusetts politics, 1900–1912* (Harvard University Press, Cambridge, Mass., 1964), p.4.

20. Barbara Rosenkrantz, *Public health and the state: changing views in Massachusetts, 1842–1936* (Harvard University Press, Cambridge, Mass., 1972), pp.74–126.

21. Neal Devitt, 'The statistical case for elimination of the midwife: fact versus prejudice, 1890–1935, part 2, *Women and Health*, vol.4 (2)

(Summer 1979), p.170.

22. *Boston Evening Globe* (8 June 1885). Letter to the Editor, 'Shall Dr. Walcott be sustained?'

23. H. R. Beecher and M. D. Aitschule, *Medicine at Harvard: the first three hundred years* (Harvard University Press, Hanover, NH, 1977), pp.92–4.

24. Abraham Flexner, *The Flexner report on medical education in the United States and Canada, 1910* (Carnegie Foundation for the Advancement of Teaching, Washington, DC, 1910, reprinted 1960), pp.117–18.

25. F. Irving, *Safe deliverance* (Houghton, Cambridge, 1942), pp.27–32.

26. *Gardner News* (17 May 1907).

27. J.P. Huntington, from his unpublished papers at the Phelps-Porter Huntington House, Hadley, Mass.

28. Register of Birth Certificates, Town Hall, Gardner, Mass., for the year 1908.

6

Nursing Power, Nursing Politics

Sidney D. Krampitz

In today's rapidly changing health care arena, a proactive position on challenges to professional integrity is a mandate. Issues of educational preparation for professional practice, credentialling for advanced clinical practice and policy decisions which control third party payment of reimbursement for nursing services confront the professional nurse of the 1980s. However, many nurses view this period not as a period of opportunity but rather from the perspective of a powerless group seeking public recognition but lacking contacts and expertise in the political area.

To the nurses of today, the controversy and opposition faced by nurses related to nurse registration and subsequent struggle to improve the status of military nurses may be lost in history. However, an understanding of the challenges facing early nurse leaders and their success in overcoming very strong opposition can inspire professional nurses of the 1980s to strive to reach new heights in education, research and practice thus insuring their permanence as key members of the health care team.

The struggle and frustration encountered by Nightingale, Dock, Wald, Goodrich and many other early nurse leaders and their remarkable vision and success can serve as an inspiration to those who seek to expand the scope of professional nursing practice. The concern for the individual patient was identified by these leaders to extend into a commitment to broad social reform issues. When one contemplates the work of Nightingale it becomes apparent that concern for the individual patient expanded to engage Nightingale with the broader concerns of the Royal Sanitary Commission, including reform in military medicine. Nightingale also clearly demonstrates concern related to creating and maintaining a healthy environment to promote wellness.[1]

However, often the rich heritage of nursing is left unexplored when current nurse leaders address issues confronting the nurse of the future. Ashley[2] and Ehrenreich and English[3] clearly document the concerted effort of American medicine in the repression of professional nursing and urged American nursing to address the inequity in the health care system.

In fact the literature is replete with examples of the devaluing of nursing education and practice by medical groups and associations. Bok[4] in *Lying: Moral Choices in Public and Private Life* explores the relationship between coercion, violence, paternalism and power and clearly identifies the role deceit plays in both coercion and paternalism. Thus both coercion and paternalism had to be addressed when early leaders sought to achieve education reform.

Professional nurses will also be required to address issues of coercion and paternalism in the decade ahead if they are to continue to serve their patients as advocates and to advance their role in the health care delivery system. Nurses must once again make a concerted effort to move from the hospital into community-based professional practice to meet the challenges of health care in the 1980s.

This chapter will focus on key issues of licensure and education in the development of American nursing, and thus has implications for nurses in their struggle to redefine professional practice in the world community of the 1980s. This struggle began in America prior to the turn of the century as expansion of hospital services to larger numbers of patients fostered the establishment of hospital training schools for nurses. The necessity of a student nurse labour force became increasingly evident to those in hospitals planning expansion and since that time the hospital has clearly had a vested interest in maintaining the status quo for nursing education and practice.

AMERICAN NURSING AND PROFESSIONALISM

The isolation of the superintendents of training schools and other nurse leaders prior to the 1890s clearly delayed the battle for registration which was to be fought a decade later. The presence of Ethel Fenwick and other British nursing leaders at the Chicago

89

World's Fair in 1893 and the papers presented at the Congress on Hospitals and Dispensaries on nurse registration, the establishment of training schools and educational standards and a professional nursing organisation clearly set the political agenda for the quarter century ahead.[5] The establishment of the American Society for Superintendents of Training Schools for Nurses shortly following the meeting speaks to the impact of British nursing on the development of professional nursing in America. The later development of the hospital economics course for graduate nurses at teachers' college and establishment of baccalaureate education for nursing in the 1920s attests to intense effort of a few on behalf of American nursing.[6] These nurses identified the establishment of a professional identity, the development of a professional organisation and the initiation of a sound educational system as essential components in the struggle to become adequately organised and academically prepared to seek public support for licensure as a profession.

Despite opposition from graduates of correspondence programmes or short-term training programmes of two to three months and selected physician groups, a broad base of well-trained nurses participated in a wide range of political activity which culminated in the passage of the first nurse practice Act in 1903. State registration has continued to be a very significant issue as a myriad of professions have sought public recognition and control of practice by establishment of restrictive licensing laws. Dock,[7] however, commented during this period that the struggle for professional registration would be ongoing. This clearly has been validated in the century which followed.

ESTABLISHING STANDARDS FOR PRACTICE

Although licensure did eliminate correspondence schools for nurses, it failed to fulfil the lofty expectations of nursing leaders. The standards which were actually established generally were based on programmes already existing in the training schools in each state and, therefore, produced neither a uniform national standard for nursing education nor a significant elevation of standards in schools of nursing.

It soon became apparent to nursing educators of that period that the establishment of state licensure, in itself, had not elevated the educational standards to the extent that these leaders had anticipated. Nurse educators and many leading physicians continued to make public appeals for broader educational preparation for nurses with little impact. It soon became imperative that nursing leaders identify alternative means to achieve the objectives of improving nursing practice and nursing education.

The conflicting goals of the delivery of patient services in the hospitals and the educational preparation of students in the hospital training school hindered the achievement of the elevated educational standards sought by nurse educators. Since the primary function of the hospital was the delivery of patient care, the training of nurses often became viewed as being merely a means of achieving this primary aim of the hospital.[8] In 1905, one prominent nurse educator, Isabel Hampton Robb, stated that although hospital authorities and superintendents had tried for some time to combine educational and service functions in a single institution, the relation of the training school to the hospital had always been an impossible one from an educational standpoint. She further charged that, until schools for nurses were founded primarily as educational institutions, the profession and the public could not hope for the establishment of uniformity in educational standards or nursing practice.[9]

Nursing leaders became increasingly concerned regarding standards in nursing education. In 1911, M. Adelaide Nutting, Chairman of the Committee on Education, American Society of Superintendents of Training Schools for Nurses, sent a letter to Henry S. Pritchett, President of the Carnegie Foundation for the Advancement of Teaching, requesting that the Foundation undertake a study of nursing education in America.[10] The Foundation had recently funded Abraham Flexner's study of medical education. Flexner's report, just published, already had made a major impact on the improvement of standards in medical education The success of the grading of medical schools stimulated the nursing community to advocate, at the 1911 annual meeting of the National League for Nursing Education, a similar grading of training schools for nurses.[11] The Carnegie Foundation was not able to support the nursing study, due to its commitment to work already initiated. However, several issues raised by Henry Pritchett of the Carnegie Foundation in his response to the Nursing Committee on Education were subsequently discussed at length by nurse educators. One of these issues was the poorly defined role of the nurse which had to be addressed before one could evaluate the existing problems in nurse training programmes.[12]

Nursing reformers, unlike reformers of medical education, were not unanimously in support of university affiliation as the means of elevating educational standards. Some leaders in medicine and nursing favoured a preliminary course for nursing students, taught in a central school;[13] others urged the closing of all schools of nursing affiliated with specialised or small hospitals.[14] While nursing leaders expressed the importance of nursing educators having college preparation, they failed to agree on a single approach to educational reform for all of nursing. The search for professional identity and the impetus for educational reform during this period of nursing history were further complicated by the fact that an evolving urban society and progressive reforms were creating a need for many highly-specialised forms of both nursing and medical care.

Many leaders in medicine and nursing during this era failed to see the tremendous needs for nursing in the area of prevention and public health. Although some 30 years earlier the first trained nurses had entered the homes of the sick poor and provided services in New York's teeming ghettos, nursing education continued to be conducted primarily in the hospital setting. When visiting nurses became affiliated with settlement houses in major industrial cities, they became acutely aware of the living standards which plagued the poor city dweller and sought relief from social problems. Klein indicates that it would be difficult to overestimate the impact of these visiting nurses on later innovations in the field of health, hygiene and medical care in America.[15]

During this same period, Lillian Wald, founder of the Henry Street Settlement, had also placed several public health nurses in New York City schools, thus demonstrating the value of the employment of nurses in the public school system. Recognising the value of this pioneer work, the Commissioner of Health appointed 12 nurses to serve New York City's school children. These community nurses became an integral part of the programme to promote health among school children. Nursing leaders became aware of the contribution which the public health nurse was capable of making and again identified the need to restructure the training of nurses to include both theory and clinical practice in the community setting.

During this period, growing pressure for political and social reform related to the changing social order fostered the expansion of the Progressive Reform Movement. Poverty, working conditions of the poor immigrant and other social issues were influenced in the final passage of the Sheppard-Towner Act in the 1920s. This Act placed emphasis on expansion of health care services to mothers and children. Smillie states that the period of 1919–29 ushered in '. . . the nationalization of the public health'.[16] The passage of legislation to improve health care for women and children also provided opportunities for the employment of public health nurses in a variety of capacities; however, the education of these nurses often was found inadequate for meeting the needs of a community-based practice and, therefore, leaders in community nursing urged university affiliation designed to provide expanded educational opportunities for nurses.[17] Changing social needs and the impact of legislation on the establishing of social programmes and educational programmes for nurses demanded a greater involvement of nurses on the political arena.

ROCKEFELLER STUDY OF NURSING AND NURSING EDUCATION

Nurse leaders were unsuccessful in their attempts to get Foundation support for a comprehensive study of nursing education in the first decade of the twentieth century. However, the growing interest of the Rockefeller Foundation in funding programmes of preventive medicine led to an interest in the newly developing field of public health nursing. Nurse leaders urged the Rockefeller Foundation to support a study of the educational preparation of nurses — a study similar to the Flexner Study of Medical Education.[18]

In 1918, the Rockefeller Foundation directors sponsored a conference for leaders in nursing and medicine to discuss problems confronting public health nursing. One outcome of this conference was a plan to conduct an investigation of the preparation of the public health nurse. This study, known as the Rockefeller Study of Nursing Education has been identified by Strong[19] and other nurse leaders as a critical step forward for nursing education. C-E. A. Winslow, Professor, Yale School of Medicine was elected Chairman of the study committee and in 1919, Josephine Goldmark, a well-recognised social scientist was appointed as a staff member with primary responsibility for the conduct of the study.

The Rockefeller Study of Nursing and Nursing Education published its final report in 1923 after several lengthy delays. However, unlike the American Medical Association Study of Nursing Education being conducted during the same period, the Rockefeller Study identified the need for broad reform in both nursing education and practice.[20,21] For example, hospital-based nurses' training demonstrated a conflict in goals between service needs and education of the student. The report states that a conflict exists in the majority of diploma nursing programmes 'between a policy of hospital administration that properly aims to care for the sick at a minimum cost, and a policy of nursing education which properly aims to concentrate a maximum of rewarding training into a minimum time'.[22]

The findings of the Rockefeller Study clearly identified the advantages of university affiliation for nursing education in contrast to the report submitted by the Committee on Trained Nursing to the Council of Medical Education of the American Medical Association, which urged university preparation for only those nurses seeking additional skills to assume management or teaching functions in specialised areas of nursing practice.[23]

In attempts at reform in nursing education, the profession always had some staunch supporters in the medical profession. However, these leaders often faced strong opposition not only from outside the medical profession but also from their medical colleagues.[24] There were those within the medical profession who were most vocal against the advancement of nursing education or the 'over-training of nurses'.[25] Individuals who favoured reform in nursing education saw the need for continued and broadened support by the medical profession if nursing education was to be improved.[26] This support came from school faculties who often identified the improvement of nursing education and practice as a means of elevating medical standards and improving medical education. This concern expressed by faculty, hospital administrators and other community leaders had broad impact on increasing public awareness of the issues involved.[27]

The relationship between nursing and medical practice was clearly becoming an issue in medical education. Hugh Cabot, Dean of the Medical School at the University of Michigan and a member of the American Medical Association Commission on Medical Education, identified nursing as 'most intimately connected with the practice of medicine . . .' He therefore asserted that, because medical practice was changing at a rate enormously greater than at any previous period in its history, 'the training of the nurse to associate herself with the practice of medicine must change at a very similar rate'.[28]

In 1931, the American Medical Association had requested that the Association's Committee on Nursing Education give consideration to the question of the relation of the AMA to nursing education. The instruction and general standards of nursing care in training schools affiliated with medical schools gained nursing much support from medical faculties in academic centres. The Committee, presenting its report in 1932 at the annual meeting of the Association of American Medical Colleges, also recognised the existing overcrowding of the nursing profession and the reluctance on the part of the most desirable candidates to enter an overcrowded profession. 'As a profession,' the report concluded, 'nurses need at least the minimum education demanded of public school teachers'.[29]

The Committee on Nursing Education of the Association of American Medical Colleges made the following recommendations: 'the influence of the School of Medicine should increasingly pervade the development of the School of Nursing'; medical schools 'should not use their nursing schools as service adjuncts of their hospitals but, if necessary, should use such additional university resources as may be necessary to bring their nursing schools up to the general level of the other colleges'; major emphasis should be placed on the development of 'adequate curriculum leading to the degree of Bachelor of Science, as well as other advanced curricula in various fields of specialized nursing endeavor'; and universities should 'accept the principle that courses in the curriculum of the school of nursing be formulated and administered with the same seriousness and on the same collegiate levels as are demanded in accredited Colleges of Arts and Sciences . . .'[30] These findings and recommendations proved to be significantly different from the early study by the American Medical Association Committee on Trained Nursing in 1922; however, appreciable change in the focus of diploma education in nursing and the expansion of baccalaureate education programmes in nursing was not seen until the 1950s. One might well raise the question as to why change did not come about. Perhaps the growing power of other parties interested in maintaining numbers of diploma nurses in the traditional hospital setting and lack of broad public support for the movement were the key issues that nurses failed to explore during this period. As a women's profession, nursing was identified as requiring dedication and sacrifice — this may have been an image of nurses more closely tied into a traditional hospital-based training programme than the education of the nurse in a university setting.

Although the findings of the Committee for the Study of Nursing Education gave some impetus to the movement of nursing education into American colleges and universities, it failed to make the impact deemed by nurse leaders as necessary to elevate standards in all of nursing education. This failure to achieve educational reform led to a proposal from the Education Committee of the National League for Nursing Education to classify or 'grade' the nursing schools of America.[31] The Education Committee proposal stated that, in the 'fields of secondary and college education, classification seems to have been equally successful in giving effectiveness to recognized standards and in stimulating public interest and support . . .' and related the substantial reform in medical education to the Flexner classification of medical schools.[32]

Many nursing and medical leaders viewed such a classification of nursing schools as a panacea for all of the problems both in hospital training schools and in those programmes having college or university affiliation. C-E. A. Winslow stated that the 'time is ripe for . . . reform' and identified the establishment of a system of grading as a means to 'make possible the gradual elimination of the poorest schools in the country and the consequent raising of the general level'.[33] The grading was to include all nursing programmes in America, as opposed to the small number of nursing programmes evaluated in the Rockefeller Study, and was designed to 'clarify' the situation in nursing education and to solicit 'public interest' in the issue of nursing standards.[34]

The Education Committee of the National League of Nursing Education developed a three-year plan for the classification of nursing schools in America. This proposal for grading schools of nursing was submitted to the Carnegie Corporation in 1923 following the completion of the Rockefeller Study of Nursing and Nursing Education. The grading study had the endorsement of all nursing, public health and hospital organisations.[35] Dean

Annie Goodrich of Yale School of Nursing stated that the study was a 'very logical result of the recent and first serious study of nursing education in the United States' and that the study was needed to correct the many shortcomings in nursing education identified in the Rockefeller Study.[36] C-E. A. Winslow, Chairman of the Rockefeller Study, endorsed the grading study and stated that there was 'no single field in education where reform is as urgently needed as that in connection with nursing education'.[37]

It was anticipated by the League that the Carnegie Corporation would support the study since the Corporation had a 'general program of improvement in hospital, medical and health work'.[38] However, the Carnegie Corporation failed to support the project, much to the chagrin of nursing leaders.[39] Determined to initiate the grading study, the professional nursing organisations provided initial financial support and appealed to other organisations, individual nurses and other private philanthropic supporters for additional resources. Initially each nursing organisation made a commitment of $10,000 to the study.[40] The study was extended from three years to five years and the cost increased from $90,000 to $200,000. Later the project was again extended to a total of seven years at a total cost of nearly $300,000.[41]

It is important to recognise that the Committee on the Grading of Nursing Schools was an outgrowth of two closely related but rather distinct issues relating to nursing and nursing education, namely, quantity and quality of nurse graduates. The primary concern on the part of many physicians was the need to increase the quantity of graduate nurses; the concern expressed most frequently by leaders in nursing and medical education, however, was the need to improve the quality of nursing education. While nursing educators were focusing on the grading study, the Medical Association was organising committees to study nursing education with a view to increasing the supply of nurses. Many of the leaders in the American Medical Association believed that it was 'more important for every patient to have some sort of nurse than a few patients to have extraordinarily good nurses . . . even if the academic standards of the schools had to be lowered to do it . . .'[42] It became imperative, in light of the concerns expressed by the Medical Association, that the grading study investigate not only the quality of nursing education but also the quantity of nurse graduates since both of

97

these issues related to nursing education and ultimately to patient care.

The Grading Committee was chaired by William Darrach, Dean, College of Physicians and Surgeons, Columbia University, who represented the American Medical Association. Initially the Grading Committee undertook a study of the supply, demand and adequacy of training nurses in America. Committee findings revealed the existence of a surplus of private duty nurses and shortage of nurses prepared in the specialty of public health nursing.[43] Findings of this study of supply and demand suggested to nursing leaders the following options:

1. Reduce and improve the supply. Make a decisive and immediate reduction in the numbers of nursing students in the United States; and raise entrance requirements high enough so that only properly qualified women will be admitted to the profession.
2. Replace students with graduates. Put the major part of the hospital bedside nursing into the hands of graduate nurses and take it out of the hands of student nurses.
3. Help hospitals meet the cost of graduate service. Assist hospitals in securing funds for the employment of graduate nurses.
4. Get public support of nursing under the direction of nurse educators instead of hospital administrators; and awaken the public to the fact that if society wants good nursing it must pay the cost of educating nurses. Nursing education is a public and not private responsibility.[44]

The oversupply of nurses in the 1920s was a result, not only of extensive recruitment efforts to meet the nursing needs during the First World War, but also of the continued development of new training schools in hospitals across the country. It is important to recognise that, during this period, few graduate nurses were employed in hospitals; the hospitals provided most of their nursing care by continually enrolling more students in their training schools. Since the new graduates were not employed by the hospitals in which they trained, they entered the overcrowded private duty nursing field. The financial depression of this period created increasing numbers of unemployed or underemployed nurses; demands for private duty nurses decreased as families could no longer provide funds for nursing services. The depression, therefore, made a significant impact on employment of graduate nurses.

However, in spite of the general overproduction of nurses, shortages of nurses did exist in some geographic areas and in certain fields of nursing. Geographic distribution was uneven with the majority of nurses living in urban areas in which they trained. This often left rural areas with acute shortages. Since few nurses had systematic preparation for executive and teaching positions in hospital or in public health nursing, there were a number of employment opportunities for such well-educated nurses.[45]

In conclusion, the first report of the Grading Committee identified the early development of hospital training schools as 'too successful' and noted that, had the training school

> cost a little more and worked a little less well, had the pioneer nurses who threw themselves into the task with such invincible enthusiasm and determination been a trifle less self-sacrificing and a bit more insistent on reasonable working hours and adequate budgets, it is probable that the nursing profession in the United States would be smaller, healthier and considerably happier.[46]

The findings and recommendations of the Grading Committee created controversy in medical and nursing organisations. While some critics focused their concern on the statistical aspects of the study, others questioned the validity of the findings and recommendations.[47] One of the concerns expressed was the possibility of creating further shortages of nurses in rural communities if the recommendations were accepted. This issue clearly related to shortages of physicians in rural areas, a problem which was created when medical schools elevated their standards with the result that fewer graduates were available to serve the public.[48]

The first grading of schools of nursing followed this initial study of supply and demand. The grading was a voluntary self-study with all schools invited to participate and assured of confidentiality. Grading was seen as one means of 'helping hospitals to improve the quality of the nursing education they are able to give . . .'[49] The grading study documented the fact that nursing education was 'dominated by some 2,000 hospital proprietary schools' and that the control of nursing education rested in hospital boards of trustees who established and maintained the schools 'because having a school is advantageous to the hospital'.[50] The study recommended: (1) that nursing education be placed on a professional basis, with responsibility for planning the courses, selecting the students and supervising their progress removed from the jurisdiction of the hospital board of trustees; (2) that educational programmes be removed from those settings in which hospitals were not equipped to educate nurses adequately; and (3) that hospitals and faculty provide for the improved utilisation of hospital clinical training opportunities.[51]

The Grading Committee brought the issue of nursing education to the public's attention but failed to solicit support on behalf of the elevation of standards in nursing education. Two hundred nursing schools were discontinued during the period of the grading and a few others affiliated with colleges or universities in an attempt to improve their basic instruction.[52] However, it is difficult to determine how many of these changes were precipitated by the grading study since a major depression during this period was influencing all sectors of the American economy. The Duke Foundation Study, completed in 1931, had demonstrated that a very small hospital could 'operate more economically without a school' and the American Nurses' Association advised superintendents of hospitals that, to 'avoid further sacrifice of quality, the traditional system of supplying the nursing services of hospitals largely by means of students in nursing schools will have to be modified considerably within the next few years'.[53] These internal and external pressures made a major impact on nursing education.

Since the Committee on the Grading of Nursing Schools had no power other than that of investigation and recommendation, it was impossible for this group to create the reorganisation essential for all nursing education to become an integral part of American higher education. Nursing leaders had anticipated that the grading study would produce a major reform in nursing education by elevating educational standards; these leaders were disappointed when the Committee proposed 'minimum standards' in its recommendations.[54] These minimum standards in admission and curriculum were already in existence in the majority of hospital training programmes and the maintenance of these standards failed to reform nursing education. The Committee agreed that existing 'schools of nursing are shockingly below the standards which they should have reached' but indicated an inability to gain public support for a radical departure from the existing hospital training.[55]

Burgess had identified two possible approaches to improving the quality of nursing education. The first option was to 'throw down the gauntlet to the medical hospital groups, to tell them that practically all their schools are bad and that they have no excuse for maintaining any of them' and that, as a result, 'the general public would turn against the medical and hospital associations and side with the nurses in order to bring these reforms about'.[56] The alternative was 'to secure the co-operation of the hospital and medical groups by approaching the problem from their viewpoint and not to reorganize everything at once but to attack only the most glaring faults and to attempt a steady campaign to pressure in the right direction, even though it may be very slow'.[57]

The existing social and political conditions of the period clearly favoured the second option. Although the public recognised the problems in nursing education, it appeared to show little 'inclination to interfere' in the existing system of nursing education and was not strongly supportive of a reorganisation of nursing education. In addition, when colleges and universities were approached regarding the establishment of nursing programmes, they indicated an interest in considering the establishment or reorganisation of a school of nursing as an integral department or school when funds were available but, 'until those funds are made available, universities will not accept the responsibility'.[58] However, when funds became available, reorganisation was undertaken in leading universities and recommendations of both the American Medical Association and the Grading Committee were evident in this reorganisation.

There appeared, at the time, to be no real prospect that nursing could indeed openly fight and win a battle for educational reform; therefore, the Grading Committee recommended the establishment of minimum educational standards and a programme of self-evaluation. This decision of the Grading Committee to avoid the classification of schools of nursing proved to be an 'exceedingly great disappointment' to nursing leaders and became a major stimulus to the development of a new organisation — the Association of Collegiate Schools of Nursing.[59]

In a 1932 address before the American Hospital Association, Burgess reported significant and 'encouraging changes'

101

following the first grading. A second grading, which had used information collected from the initial evaluation, demonstrated improvement in standards in nursing education and more constructive relationships between medical-hospital-nursing groups as these groups focused on 'active experimentation in solving nursing problems'.[60]

One major recommendation of the Grading Committee was the establishment of a National Council on Nursing and Nursing Education which would 'stimulate, protect, and guide the developments in professional nursing'.[61] This recommendation was intended to involve both nursing and medical professions in joint planning for the further development of nursing as the Grading Committee identified support from the medical profession as essential to initiate reform in education. However, the proposed National Council was never established and the responsibility for continued reform in nursing education became a function of professional nursing groups — in particular the National League of Nursing Education. This aborted effort at co-operative planning was similar to the brief dialogue on practice between nursing and medicine that followed the National Commission Study of Nursing and Nursing Education of the 1970s. In addition to the failure of the National Council to materialise, the 'practical handbook' which was to be the final publication of the Grading Committee and was to be used as 'a tool for the grading by local and national organizations' also failed to be developed, leaving the nursing profession with another extensive study which did not achieve its goal.[62]

The success and failure of these early nursing leaders in their attempts at reform can shed light on the barriers and issues which must be addressed in the entry into practice controversy and the political and social dynamics which continue to drive nursing education in the 1980s. Obviously licensure and the establishment of a minimal standard is not the issue today; however, the political forces and lack of public support remain as a barrier to expanded professional practice.

In concluding, nurse leaders can clearly gain a perspective as they address the challenges ahead by assessing the imperfect past for a lesson for the future. Political awareness and active participation in the political arena are essentials in the nursing profession's efforts to influence public opinion and public policy as the profession seeks to better serve its students and its public. The past has taught us all lessons that we must not forget.

NOTES

1. C. Woodham-Smith, *Florence Nightingale* (Constable, London, 1953).

2. J. Ashley, *Hospitals, paternalism and the role of the nurse* (Teachers' College Press, New York, 1976).

3. B. Ehrenreich and D. English, *Witches, midwives and nurses: a history of women healers* (The Feminist Press, New York, 1973).

4. S. Bok, *Lying: moral choice in public and private life* (Vintage Books, New York, 1979).

5. L. Dock, *A history of nursing* (Putnams, New York, 1935), Vol. 3.

6. S. Krampitz, 'Historical development of baccalaureate nursing education in American nursing, 1895–1935', doctoral dissertation, University of Chicago, 1978.

7. L. Dock, 'State registration', *American Journal of Nursing* (AJN),2 (September 1902), pp.979–85.

8. 'Proceedings of the Fifth Annual Convention of the Nurses' Associated Alumnae of the United States', *AJN*, 2 (July 1902), pp.747–51; 'Minutes of the proceedings, Sixth Annual Convention of the Nurses' Associated Alumnae of the United States, 1903', AJN, 3 (August 1903), p.840; and 'Editor's miscellany', *AJN*, 3 (September 1903), pp.996–7.

9. I. H. Robb, *Educational standards for nurses* (Koechert, Cleveland, 1907), pp.223–45.

10. M. A. Nutting to H. S. Pritchett, 10 June 1911, Archives of the Department of Nursing Education, File 2, Drawer 2, Folder: Carnegie Foundation, Teachers' College, Columbia University, New York (Dept of Nursing Education Archives)

11. A. Flexner, *Medical education in the United States and Canada: a report to the Carnegie Foundation for the advancement of teaching* (Merrymount Press, Boston, Mass., 1910).

12. H. S. Pritchett to M. A. Nutting, 17 June 1911, Dept of Nursing Education Archives.

13. M. A. Nutting, 'The preliminary education of nurses', *AJN*, 1 (March 1901), pp.416–24; M. J. Hurdley, 'How can training schools best co-operate with existing educational institutions?', in *Proceedings of the Eighteenth Annual Convention of the American Society of Superintendents of Training Schools for Nurses* (Thatchery Art Printery, Springfield, Mass., 1912), pp.26–30; and S. M. Weir, 'Nurses and their education', *AJN*, 2 (August 1902), pp.899–909.

14. L. R. Logan, 'A program for the grading of schools of nursing', *AJN*, 25 (December 1925), p.1005.

15. P. Klein, *From philanthropy to social welfare: an american cultural perspective* (Jossey-Bass, San Francisco, 1968), p.116.

16. W. G. Smillie, *Preventive medicine and public health* (Macmillan, New York, 1952), 2nd edn, p.10.

17. 'Report of the Committee on Nursing Education' (22 June 1922), pp.2–3, Dept of Nursing Education Archives.

18. Flexner, *Medical education*.

19. A.H. Strong, 'The nursing situation from the public health point

of view', *Transactions of the American Hospital Association*, pp.302–8.

20. *Committee on the Study of Nursing Education, Nursing and Nursing Education in the United States: report of the committee* (Macmillan, New York, 1923), pp.97–106.

21. 'Preliminary report of the Committee on Trained Nursing to the Council of Medical Education and Hospitals of American Medical Association', typescript (1902), p.7, Dept of Nursing Education Archives.

22. 'Report of the Committee on Nursing Education' (22 June 1922), pp.2–3, Dept of Nursing Education Archives.

23. 'Preliminary Report of the Committee on Trained Nurses', pp.19–24.

24. Dr George Walker introduced a Bill into the 1935 Maryland legislature to force nurses to have a college education and to place nursing under state supervision. He appeared alone against 500 opponents at a committee hearing and went down in defeat; see 'Dr. George Walker', *The Sun* (1 April 1937), Dept of Nursing Education Archives.

25. I. M. Stewart, 'Developments in nursing education since 1918', *Bulletin 1921*, no.20, Department of the Interior, Bureau of Education, p.18, Archives Nursing Collection, Box 120, Folder: Nursing Collegiate Relationships, Sterling Library, Yale University, New Haven (Nursing Collection Archives). See also May Ayres Burgess to Dr Frank Billings, 18 October 1926, Dept of Nursing Education Archives.

26. M. A. Burgess, 'Three problems of nurses', *Proceedings, Congress on Medical Education, Licensure, Public Health and Hospitals, Chicago, February 1928* (reprint) p.11, Nursing Collection Archives.

27. C. W. Munger, 'The school committee and the hospital ward', *Annual Report, 1935, and Proceedings of the National League of Nursing Education Forty-First Convention* (The League, New York, 1935), pp.134–6; George Walker to Adelaide Nutting, 4 October 1933, Dept of Nursing Education Archives.

28. H. Cabol, 'The role of the university in nursing education', *Annual Report, 1928, and Proceedings of the National League of Nursing Education Thirty-Fourth Convention* (The League, New York, 1928), p.199.

29. 'Report of the Committee on Nursing Education', *Journal of the Association of American Medical Colleges*, 88 (January 1933), p.28.

30. Ibid., pp.38–9. See also E. P. Lyons, 'The concern of the medical school in nursing education', *Annual Report, 1933, and Proceedings of the National League of Nursing Education Thirty-Ninth Convention* (The League, New York, 1933).

31. National League of Nursing Education, minutes of the board of directors (17 June 1923), Nursing Collection Archives.

32. E. J. Taylor, 'Proposed plan for the classification of nursing schools' (13 February 1923), Nursing Collection Archives.

33. C-E. A. Winslow to B. S. Quinn (sic), Assistant Director, Commonwealth Fund (20 November 1924), Archive, Department of Public Health, Box 7, Folder: C-E. A. Winslow, Sterling Library, Yale University, New Haven (Dept of Public Health Archives).

34. Taylor, 'Proposed plan for the classification of nursing schools'.

35. B. S. Quin to A. W. Goodrich, 18 November 1924, Nursing Collection Archives.

36. A. W. Goodrich to B. S. Quinn (sic), 9 December 1924, Nursing Collection Archives.

37. C-E. A. Winslow to B. S. Quinn (sic), 20 November 1924, Nursing Collection Archives.

38. E. J. Taylor to A. W. Goodrich, 13 February 1933, Nursing Collection Archives.

39. Minutes of the joint meeting of the board of directors, ANA, NLNE and NOPHN (23 April 1925) (summary), Nursing Collection Archives.

40. C. M. Hall, 'Report on the Nurses' Committee for Financing the Grading Plan, *Annual Report, 1927, and Proceedings of the National League of Nursing Education Thirty-Third Convention* (The League, New York, 1927), p.60.

41. Committee on the Grading of Nursing Schools, *Nursing schools today and tomorrow: final report of the Committee on the Grading of Nursing Schools* (The Committee, New York, 1934), p.17. Mrs Helen Hartley Jenkins had supported nursing education earlier at Teachers' College, Columbia University; see Chapter II. See also 'Financial report: Executive Committee of the Committee on the Grading of Nursing Schools' (14 November 1927), Dept of Public Health Archives; The Rockefeller Foundation, minutes of the board of directors, meeting of 10 June 1927, Foundation Archives, 200 C Committee on the Grading of Nursing Schools 1926–1929, RG 1.1, Series 200, Box 121, Folder 1492, The Rockefeller Foundation Archives, North Tarrytown, New York (Rockefeller Archives).

42. M. A. Burgess, 'Plans and Budgets for a five year program submitted to the committee on the grading of nursing schools' (18 November 1926), Dept of Public Health Archives.

43. Dr W. Darrach and Dr C-E. A. Winslow were staunch supporters of the elevation of standards in nursing education. Dr Darrach was appointed as member-at-Large and continued his participation in the study when the American Medical Association withdrew its support. M. A. Burgess, *Nurses, patients and pocketbooks: report of a study of the economics of nursing conducted by the Committee on the grading of Nursing Schools* (The Committee, New York, 1928), p.iii. See also 'Report of the Committee on the Grading of Nursing Schools', *Annual Report, 1925, and Proceedings of the National League of Nursing Education Thirty-First Convention* (The League, New York, 1925), p.58.

44. M. A. Burgess, 'Nurses, patients and pocketbooks', *Trained Nurse and Hospital Review*, 81 (July 1928), p.69.

45. Committee on the Grading of Nursing Schools, 'Nurses' production, education, distribution and pay', n.d., Nursing Collection Archives.

46. M. A. Burgess, 'Committee on the Grading of Nursing Schools', (manuscript) (20 November 1928) Dept of Public Health Archives.

47. A. C. Sutton, 'The Grading Committee's report: analysis by a

statistician', *Trained Nurse and Hospital Review*, 81 (November 1928), pp.559–61.

48. B. C. Smith, General Director, Commonwealth Fund, to C-E. A. Winslow, 12 December 1928, Dept of Public Health Archives. See also Barry C. Smith to William Darrach, Chairman, Committee on the Grading of Nursing Schools, 4 December 1928, Dept of Public Health Archives.

49. M. A. Burgess, 'The first grading', *AJN*, 29 (April 1929), p.4 (reprint), Special Collections Department, Vanderbilt University School of Nursing, Box 12, Folder 10: W. W. Leathers, 1924–29, Joint University Libraries, Nashville.

50. M. A. Burgess to E. Taylor, 17 February 1931, Nursing Collection Archives.

51. Ibid.

52. O. Pecord, 'The Future of nursing schools', *Trained Nurse and Hospital Review*, 86 (May 1931), p.654.

53. American Nurses' Association, Committee on the Distribution of Nursing Service, to Hospital Superintendents, 2 July 1932, Dept of Nursing Education Archives.

54. A. Goodrich to M. A. Burgess, 21 March 1932, Nursing Collection Archives.

55. M. A. Burgess to A. Goodrich, 25 March 1932, Nursing Collection Archives.

56. Ibid.

57. Ibid.

58. Ibid.

59. Ibid.

60. M. A. Burgess, 'Quality nursing' (typescript) (15 September 1932), Nursing Collection Archives.

61. M. A. Burgess to the Committee on the Grading of Nursing Schools, 30 November 1932, p.32, Nursing Collection Archives.

62. 'The Grading Committee plans', *The Trained Nurse and Hospital Review*, 88 (January 1932), p.54. Although funding for the publication of the final report and handbook had been received from the Rockefeller Foundation, Dr Burgess was unable to complete the proposed handbook. See the following documents located in the Rockefeller Archives — minutes of the executive committee, meeting of 15 January 1932.

The Emergence of Training Programmes for Asylum Nursing at the Turn of the Century*

Olga Maranjian Church

As an emerging group from within nursing, psychiatric nursing was claimed as a segment[1] *after* it had served in apprenticeship programmes developed by psychiatrists. Thus, organised nursing proclaimed the mission, defined the work roles and relationships and created associations to forward the interest of this speciality group three decades after the first organised psychiatrist-initiated programme was established in 1882.

The history of this occupational group's efforts to assume the status of a profession is very much related to this documentation of the movement and evolution of psychiatric nursing as it accumulated those attributes that designate a profession, that is, as it developed out of a state of apprenticeship toward an autonomous and self-reliant discipline.

From the work of the early alienists,[2] who sought to provide care for the inmates of asylums, to the educational options developed by pioneering nurses, such as those at the Johns Hopkins Training School, the study presented here provides a glimpse of the emergence of psychiatric training programmes at the turn of the century.

Individual attempts at lunacy reform early in the nineteenth century had neither successfully transformed the attitudes of the general population nor made inroads in the traditional custodial approach. Though the rhetoric by the mid-nineteenth century implied a genteel and morally right rehabilitation, the reality identified by reformers such as Dorothea Dix revealed harsh

* Olga Maranjian Church, 'Emergence of Training Programmes for Asylum Nursing at the Turn of the Century', *Advances in Nursing Science: Nursing History Edition*, vol.7, no.2 (January 1985), pp.35–46. Reprinted with permission of Aspen Publishers, Inc.

treatments and the persistent view that mental alienation was a hopelessly dehumanising process rendering its deranged victims insensitive and irreversibly damaged.

Social reformers as well as alienists in the medical community continued to be concerned about the need for developing caretakers for physically and mentally ill citizens. Such concern is visible in the public records. For example, in 1850, the Sanitary Commissioners of the State of Massachusetts recommended:

> that institutions be formed to educate and qualify females to be nurses of the sick . . . Bad nursing often defeats the intentions of the best medical advice and good nursing often supplies the defects of bad advice. Nursing often does more to cure disease than the physician himself; and in the prevention of disease and in the promotion of health it is of equal and even greater importance.[3]

Though these Commissioners, presumably all men, were anxious to recruit women for such work, the appropriate sphere for women of the nineteenth century continued to be in the home.

Ultimately, women willing to do good works entered nursing first and most dramatically during the Civil War but in a sustained and organised fashion during the Reconstruction Period. At about the same time, news of the accomplishments and publications of Florence Nightingale became available in the United States. Prior to this, schools for training nurses established by and for physicians were already firmly entrenched throughout the populated areas of the nation.

By 1873, the Nightingale system of training was officially adopted in the United States by the establishment of three schools within a one-year period. The first, the Bellevue Training School for nurses, opened in New York in May. This system provided a certain amount of autonomy for the programmes and allowed administrative independence from the hospitals in which the students were trained. With some modification it was:

> 'based on Miss Nightingale's uncompromising doctrine that all control over the nursing staff' as to selection, discipline, rotation in hospital wards, and standards of teaching, of ethics and of morals, 'should be placed in the hands of the Matron or Superintendent, who must herself be a trained nurse,' and

responsible to the hospital and medical authorities for the faithful carrying out of medical orders and institutional regulations.[4]

By October 1873, the Connecticut Training School opened at the New Haven Hospital and the following month, the Boston Training School at the Massachusetts General Hospital followed suit.[5] Both of these programmes were under the management of committees of men and women who served on special training school boards.

By the late nineteenth century, a few alienists in the vanguard of reform in the treatment of lunacy identified the need for specialised training of asylum care-takers. The protagonist in the development of what was to become asylum nursing was Dr Edward Cowles. He was responsible for opening 'the first formally organized training school within a hospital for the insane in the world'[6] at the McLean Asylum in Waverly, Massachusetts, in 1882. By this time, McLean already had a long and interesting history, being the first hospital built in the state of Massachusetts. 'The need to house the insane, seen as more urgent than a general hospital by the Massachusetts General Hospital Corporation, which functioned under a charter by the state legislature',[7] had resulted in the opening of the McLean Asylum in 1818, three years before the Massachusetts General Hospital opened for general patient care.

Cowles, who became Superintendent of McLean in 1879, established the nurse training programme as part of a campaign to 'medicalise' the asylum. Determined to alter the image as well as the approach in the care of the mentally alienated, he proclaimed that attendants would become 'nurses' and inmates would become 'patients'. He was responsible for removing bars from windows, experimenting with unlocked doors and admitting visitors without imposing restrictions.[8]

The shift to *nursing* the mentally alienated was essential to his efforts in medicalising the asylum. Cowles explained that:

The word 'attendant' is unfortunate, although it is so much better than the older term, 'keeper'. It would be only the truth to call them 'nurses' . . . the idea of the hospital is in it all, and no attempt should be made to ignore it. It should appear rather that active attention is being given to the business of curing the sick. 'Attendants' may attend the infirm and incur-

109

able; but 'nurses' attend the sick, and the experience of recovery from illness is so common that the very presence of a nurse logically carries with it the other idea, that something is being done to promote recovery, and that itself inspires hope and is curative. The key note of all that is addressed to the patient on this subject should be *you* are ill, you may get well.[9]

Cowles maintained that women, given their natural capabilities for nurturance, in their role as nurses, provided great beneficial value to the inmates, who were to be considered patients. Ten years later, under his direction, the asylum was officially renamed the McLean Hospital. Thus, medicalisation of the asylum became possible through training asylum nurses, and Cowles as the foremost physician in nursing reform for the insane sought to inspire his colleagues to follow his example.

Prior to his arrival at McLean, Cowles briefly served as superintendent at the Boston City Hospital. While there, 'with the assistance of Miss Linda Richards, the first American woman in the United States to hold a diploma as a trained nurse', he began the Training School for Nurses at the Boston City Hospital, '. . . the first in the United States that was part of the hospital organization itself, and independent of outside assistance'.[10] This organisational structure was *not* in keeping with the Nightingale system, and, as such, serves as an early indicator of the domination of and influence on nurse training programmes by hospital administrators and physicians.

Although Cowles spoke favourably about Nightingale as the 'founder of Modern Nursing', he avoided following her basic principle of autonomy in his establishment of the training programmes both at Boston City and at McLean. He spoke often of nursing and Nightingale as responsible for 'that Noble Reform'; he said that 'no greater work has ever been done for the amelioration of human suffering and saving of human life than this . . .', and he credited Nightingale with the '. . . creation of an epoch for the hospitals while the asylums were still groping to find the way in which they first felt the need of going'.[11]

In 1887, he acknowledged the difficulties in the initiation of such a movement:

In 1873 the instructed nurse was an experiment, and a cause of apprehension. It was said she would know too much, or would think that she need not obey the physician in all particulars;

she would tamper with the treatment; she would want to be a doctor herself, etc. Now there are in this country, few general hospitals of importance in which nurses are not carefully trained in their duties, according to well established methods of instructions.[12]

In his public and private remarks Cowles persisted in his belief that schools should teach the skills of both physical and mental nursing. He firmly believed that preparing students for 'bodily' as well as 'mental' nursing would allow the student to be more versatile in future endeavours. Predicting that the 'specialist nurse' would be a failure, his approach anticipated the complications that ultimately evolved in speciality education of nurses and the various efforts to integrate the nursing student's experiences. Ultimately, affiliation programmes were established in which asylum students served a certain amount of time studying and practising various aspects of general nursing.

In 1887, while assessing the progress of his reform, Cowles acknowledged the special 'undesirable' character of asylum nursing service and spoke of the work as 'repulsive' and 'trying'.[13] The ideal attendant was one with religious motives, a cultivated mind and a benevolent heart. But he emphasised that the ideal *could not* be realised unless and until the asylums applied the obvious 'business principles' that had made it possible for general hospital programmes to succeed. He maintained that:

> The asylums, all the time, begin at the wrong end of the problem, ignoring too much the larger view. The limited object of the immediate interests of the service, and of the insane in the asylums, the ease of giving a few lectures which made a quick but deceptive show of 'systematic training', the lack of the sustaining, moral and business force of the outside organizations by which the first training schools were established in the hospitals have led to disappointment and failure. The warning is plain; the lesson is — lay a good foundation for your work and build upon it safely and surely.[14]

He also pointed out that 'another of the prime causes of the failures was that no public demand had been created for asylum-trained nurses'.[15] In discussing how such public demand for the special skills of asylum nurses might be stimulated, Cowles clarified his priorities of the asylum school programme. Acquiring the true asylum spirit was paramount to the training of successful nurses. The initial question was:

> How shall we make a nurse that will be useful to the public and command its patronage; in other words, how shall we best subserve the grand purpose of all our work, the public good, to which the general interest of the nurse is incidental and complemental, and really a means to a greater good?[16]

Cowles's solution was to provide a firm foundation of general nursing skills in the first year of training, to which special mental nursing skills could be added. Thus, the students acquired 'the professional spirit that animates good work in that field, besides gaining some satisfactory practical knowledge of this business'.[17] The importance of selecting appropriate candidates for asylum work was carefully considered, and Cowles spoke of the natural talents of women as opposed to men, in this field. Although he was to begin one of the first such organised training programmes for men in 1886, his caution in the use of men as nurses was grounded in the idea that men 'do not lend themselves so pliably as women to the spirit of the work'.[18]

Speaking of the risk involved in teaching women who might be misguided into thinking of themselves as more than nurses, Cowles referred to women who sought honest and respectable livelihoods and who had no 'higher motives'. He acknowledged the misgivings of the medical community at large, and referred to 'timely caution . . . against training the woman so that she becomes a sort of hybrid, which is neither nurse nor doctor'.[19] He reassured his colleagues that:

> At the McLean Asylum the nurses are not taught to write theses and the like; they are quietly handed their diplomas when they are due, and there is rigid avoidance of promoting any other spirit than that of aiming at modest, quiet, unobtrusive devotion to honest work.[20]

Cowles often spoke of 'two maxims that apply to the well-instructed nurse: "The more you trust, the more you may", and "People generally do what you expect of them".'[21] Basically, he determined that:

What was wanted in the nurse was intelligence, sympathy, and trustworthiness. It was seen that the secret of Florence Nightingale's success was in overcoming repugnance to the work of nursing by giving the nurse better knowledge of the nature of disease and how to relieve suffering. The natural motherliness of the nurse was at once enlisted by teaching her what to do. This aroused and awakened the sympathy of intelligent minds, and thus came character and trustworthiness. For the insane, it was only necessary to apply the same principle.[22]

Cowles was unusual in his faith in the acute intuition of women as nurses. Most physicians of the nineteenth century, seen by society as the guardians of morality,[23] were concerned with women's proper place, and publicly debated this issue. Ostensibly discussing the appropriate preparation for entry into nursing, many physicians discussed the dangers of the physical and moral weakness of women. That physicians should control and be instructors in the 'art and science of nursing', was considered appropriate and in keeping with the self-appointed authority that had been proclaimed earlier.

Many, but not all, of the nineteenth-century alienists were practising 'moral management'. This treatment modality, first established in the late eighteenth century, was aimed at correcting and controlling the social, psychological and physical components of the patient and the environment. Moral management implied that the patient's condition was a direct result of immorality, i.e. that some inherent moral or sinful weakness needed to be corrected. Therefore, the proper management of a patient's life would make it possible for redemption and rehabilitation.

The alienists wrote on the subject of 'nervous' (asylum) nursing and held decided opinions and 'grave concerns' of the dangers if a nurse should attempt to advance herself through education or inappropriate training. The fear was that:

The nurse, by endeavoring to advance, might exceed her sphere; that in attempting to do better, she would do more too much, perhaps — unsexing herself by attempting all the duties of the opposite sex, for many of which, at certain times, she is physiologically unfitted, and on the other, injuring the patient by excessive kindness or mistaken zeal.[24]

For the most part, arguments were based on biological determination. Underlying the concerns about misconduct in the guise of patient care was the issue of inherent physiological problems of being female. Identified as such, this became the vital inescapable and legitimate proof against women in the workplace and was generalised and validated by the moralist/ alienist who spoke out.

General nursing's first organisational efforts did not surface until the World's Columbian Exposition in 1893 in Chicago. The idea of an association for nurses developed at the meeting of the subsection on nursing of the International Congress of Charities, Correction and Philanthropy. The work of the nurse, the preparation to do such work and the need to develop a code of ethics and standards in nursing education were issues of great concern discussed by the nurses in attendance, many of whom were nursing superintendents. This group later decided to establish the Society of Superintendents of Training Schools for Nurses of the United States and Canada,[25] which was one of the first professional women's groups to organise on a national basis.

It is ironic that at the nurses' conference, a paper was presented that described a brief history of the care of the insane and offered a summary of the state of the art in 1893.[26] In the discussion that followed, the only question recorded was one that raised concern regarding the credibility of calling an asylum a hospital and an attendant a nurse. The speaker's response was, 'I never call an attendant a nurse myself . . .'[27] Both the question and the response underscore the separate arenas of care, i.e. the hospital and the asylum. It seems the nurses in attendance at the conference had yet to identify the similarities as clearly as they had the differences in the work involved in each.

At the same international gathering in Chicago, there was a meeting of the International Congress of Charities, Corrections and Philanthropy dealing with commitment, detention and care and treatment of the insane. In attendance, in addition to many social scientists and educators, were the members of the American Medico-Psychological Association. The President, Dr J. B. Andrews, discussed the issue of training asylum nurses as an element of progress.

> The proposition to substitute nurses instead of jailors, guards or attendants in the care of the insane, seems so simple and rational that we are astonished that only during the last

quarter of the nineteenth century has it been put into form and practice. When this was once recognized in a practical way by the establishment of training schools for nurses of the insane, it immediately attracted universal attention and received general approval . . . We have passed the period of experiment and may now formulate a more complete and perfect system. The subject is of such importance to all that I would suggest the propriety of the appointment, by the Association, of a committee to prepare a definite scheme and, so far as possible, a uniform method of procedure for asylum training schools. The advantages to be gained by such action are so apparent that I need not enumerate them.[28]

The advantages of more and better trained nurses did not inspire the Association members to move on Andrews's suggestion.[29] It was another 13 years of annual meetings before the membership appointed such a committee. The irony of similar concerns, expressed by physicians and nurses with regard to regulation and standardisation of training programmes, at the same place, during the same conference, with seemingly no regard for one another's involvement, is apparent. Yet the newly emerging organised group of nurses was in no position to take on the responsibility of asylum training, for they had yet to organise the most fundamental core of education for the practice of traditional nursing. As a separate area of concern for nursing, asylum training would have to wait.

In spite of such neglect and influenced by the 'common sense' of the sociocultural considerations in approaching patient care, some of the early nursing leaders did include the wider realm of mental health in the rhetoric and the definition of the scope of nursing practice. They recognised the importance of prevention and the need for public involvement in health education; yet, the acceptance of their ideas and suggestions was impeded by social and economic factors as well as by circumstances from within and outside nursing proper.

The background of the World's Fair provided an atmosphere of promise and progress in the newly urbanised industrial society and was an appropriate setting for this inspired group of women. Nursing pioneers at the Chicago World's Fair were aware of their potential impact on the health care of the nation. No longer was nursing to be limited to the private homes of the wealthy for private duty. Nursing was emerging with a professional commitment to a public responsibility.

In 1906, at the annual meeting of the American Medico-Psychological Association, papers discussed the value of training the attendants and nurses in asylums. Implicit in the issues was the need for involvement of the medical superintendents in the training that was offered. Papers entitled 'The Male Nurse', 'Night Nurses for the Insane', 'The Training School in the Insane Hospital', and 'Musings Concerning Nurses in Hospitals for the Insane' were presented.[30]

This Symposium on Nursing included a lengthy discussion following on the formal presentations. An interesting issue was whether men or women would make better companions for male patients. One argument offered that:

> When men patients want to go to the theatre, play ball, go to the city, etc., the competent male nurses can go with them, which women nurses could not do properly . . . If good trained men are not to be obtained, we may have to rely on trained women attendants upon the male patients, but where the good men can be obtained, and can be well instructed . . . they should be the responsible caretaker of the majority of men patients . . . If women are in responsible charge of men, you only get an inferior grade of men, who will be willing to take the irresponsible and degrading subordinate positions.[31]

Thus, the underlying issue was not the competence of the female nurses in patient care; rather, the concerns rested on the impact of female nurses being 'in charge' of male attendants and male nurses. Cowles, in attendance at this meeting, discussed the advantages of both male and female nurses. He referred to 'certain fundamental principles', and 'that there must be some underlying reason for the difficulty that had existed for half a century in the many attempts that had been made to train attendants for the insane'.[32] Identifying the fundamental principle as one based on a fair exchange of goods and services, Cowles explained that if you wanted the nurses, male or female, to do things for you, you would have to do something for them.

> The principle of the establishment of training schools was a recognition of the practical fact that nurses ought to receive that which would repay them for giving their services to the hospital . . . It is easily determined that they must be given a

profession, and be attracted to the hospital for the insane by a like fair return for their service . . . With men, it is a more difficult question . . . Some equivalent must be given to the men as to the women, either in the way of education or of compensation as wages.[33]

The qualities of both male and female applicants were discussed fully, with all agreeing that special requirements for nursing the insane included special material out of which to make such nurses. The general sentiment expressed was that:

The amount of intelligence, tact, judgement and skill required to care properly for an insane person is infinitely greater than that required to care properly for even a surgical patient in a general hospital. There is need of missionary work with the public to teach the importance of intelligent care of the insane.[34]

Perhaps the most telling remarks from this meeting speak to the stereotypic image of the nurse as the essence of 'pure, sweet woman'. Those in attendance warned that:

The more gentle and womanly, the better the nurse. Now as the woman becomes a little mannish, as is the tendency of the present day, she spoils her usefulness as a nurse. The best male nurse is effeminate and is good accordingly as he approaches a woman in his characteristics.[35]

In closing the Symposium on Nursing, Dr W. A. White made the motion that was suggested by Andrews 13 years earlier, the motion to appoint a committee:

To be known as the Committee on Training Schools, whose duty shall be to prescribe a minimum requirement in a course of study in training schools for nurses in hospitals for the insane and that the diplomas issued by those hospitals in the judgement of the committee, satisfy the requirements, and shall be accepted in other hospitals for the insane. The motion was duly seconded and carried.[36]

The first report from that Committee was submitted at the next annual meeting and was accepted and adopted by the Association on 8 May 1907. Included in this report was the disclaimer that if the course work suggested by the committee seemed too advanced to the association members, they should consider that 'with the advance of recent years in the care and treatment of the sick the minimum of what a nurse should know cannot be small'.[37]

Thus it was that a group of five physicians, having been duly appointed by their fellow alienists and having consulted with superintendents of Training Schools for Nurses in Hospitals for the Insane, determined the candidates and the context to be taught in the asylum training programmes.[38] They defined the major function of the nurse as 'to assist the physician in the care of his patients' and determined that:

> assistance to the physician in the care and treatment of the insane is greater, more important and calls for a higher service than in any other form of disease, and the need for careful instruction and training is correspondingly greater . . . In order that this assistance and service may be intelligent there is need of instruction similar in kind to that of the physician, though differing in degree.[39]

This last comment regarding the difference as one of degree was unfortunate, as it implied that nurses and physicians not only have the need for the same information but also have the same orientation in carrying out their individual missions. There was no consideration for a difference in approach or scope of care, merely one of degree. If this was a generalised sentiment on the part of the physicians, then it is understandable that any educational advances for nurses could be perceived as a threat and that the appropriation of control over how much a nurse should know would serve the best interests of those so threatened.

The powerful influence of the curative/medical model on the evolution of psychiatric nursing and the current acknowledgement of the limitations of such a model have given rise to recent challenges and a growing rejection of this ideology. Medicine as disease and treatment oriented held a narrow focus. Nursing's basic orientation from its inception traditionally included disease prevention and health promotion in its scope of concern.

The American Psychiatric Association's first Committee on Training Schools for Nurses marks the official assumption of control of the practice of mental nursing by this organisation. After establishing standards and submitting its report by 1907, the Committee remained inactive until 1918, when once again the need to assert control over the 'problem' of asylum nursing was demonstrated. Another such committee was then appointed on a permanent basis and functioned until the mid 1950s.

Asylum nursing would be part of the newly recognised clinical field of psychopathology and, for a brief period during the first few decades of this century, was referred to as 'psychopathic' nursing. Though the dichotomy between the physical and mental aspects of illness prevailed, recognition of the arbitrary nature in dealing with nursing care in such a manner was not lost on nursing's pioneers in education and psychiatry.

For example, Effie J. Taylor, the first nursing director of the Phipps Clinic at Johns Hopkins Hospital, developed the first general hospital course offering training for nurses in psychiatric care. Taylor's pioneering programme, in place when the Phipps opened its doors in 1913, had as its main objective the integration of basic concepts from general and mental nursing. Her ultimate aim was to establish a comprehensive knowledge base from which all nursing could emanate.

Taylor sought to expand the scope of nursing education so there would be no arbitrary division of patient mind and body and so the student experience would lead to the synthesis of all learning throughout the programme. Taylor's wisdom in this regard is evident in her many comments on the educational advantages of viewing the patient as a whole. She maintained that 'there is no such thing as mental nursing apart from general nursing or general nursing apart from mental nursing'[40]; the course of study she developed was based on this concept of the 'oneness' of the whole being. She emphasised the value of such a programme and the opportunity at the clinic for student growth and understanding.

It is in this, and in the fact also that opportunity is given the pupil nurses in their regular course to establish firmly in their minds that physical and mental illness must be studied together, and are each an equally important part of their professional education, that the hope of the future rests.[41]

The three decades that spanned the time between Cowles's asylum training programme and the educational offering established by Taylor were decades of rapid developments, with reforms in education and social welfare. Cowles's 'programme' emerged from an identified need for service. Taylor's programme was part of a firmly established and prominent training school at an internationally recognised medical centre. Taylor continued her concern for broadening the base of nurse education in subsequent efforts at Yale University (New Haven, Connecticut) where she was appointed 'the world's first professor of psychiatric nursing', and in 1934 she succeeded Annie W. Goodrich and became the second dean at the school of nursing.

Psychiatric nursing reform from within proceeded very slowly. Organisational support for surveys and committees on the care of the insane provided some insight into the largely unexplored arena where few 'trained' nurses ventured. However, official recognition of its growing importance is demonstrated by the inclusion of 'nursing in mental and nervous diseases' in all three curriculum guides developed and distributed in 1917 and 1937 by the National League for Nursing Education.

By the mid-1930s, along with the passage of social security legislation, which was the first overt indication of Federal government support for nursing education, there was an escalation in organised nursing activities with regard to psychiatric nursing. The National League for Nursing Education developed suggested course outlines for postgraduate work in psychiatric nursing, and more surveys, reports and committees ultimately led to collaboration between organised nursing and organised psychiatry. In retrospect, it is clear that progress would be limited.

Though much occurred in the social arena during the first four decades of this century, the role of the trained nurse in improving conditions for psychiatric care remained restricted to the prevailing medical ideology. The development of a scientifically and academically broader perspective for nursing was complicated by differences based on sex, ideology and discipline. The physicians, some sympathetic, others paternalistic, and many exploitive, continued in their authoritative control of the psychiatric setting. As long as the work of the mental nurse was confined to the mental institutions, the role was likewise restricted. Once nursing education programmes ventured beyond the institutional walls into the educational mainstream of academia, such restrictions were considerably diminished.

The rhetoric from the turn of the century implied direct involvement in patient care and management of the therapeutic environment as the psychiatric nurse's responsibility. The expansion of the nurse's role into the arena of *mental health*, as opposed to that limited to *mental illness*, had been envisioned by articulate nursing pioneers. But for almost half a century, the essential divergence from the restrictive focus of the medical model was all but impossible to achieve.

Widespread governmental intervention supporting preventive measures and promotion of health education beginning with the Mental Health Act of 1946 finally legitimised the expanded role of what has become psychiatric-mental health nursing and released it from medical domination. Once society and in particular the medical profession seriously examined the restrictive nature of the boundaries that defined deviance as mental disease, the therapeutic tyranny of the medical model was greatly reduced. As the social definition of psychiatric care increasingly encompassed mental health concerns on a community-wide basis, the care-taking role of the nurse correspondingly expanded to accomodate these concerns.

NOTES

1. Segment defined as '. . . groupings of professionals that share both an organized identity and a common professional fate'.; R. Butcher, 'Pathology: a study of social movements within a profession' *Soc. Probl.*, vol 10 (1962), pp.40–51.

2. Mental alienation was the commonly used term in the nineteenth and twentieth centuries to designate mental illness and the early psychiatrists were known as alienists.

3. L. Shattuck, *Report of the Sanitary Commission of Massachusetts, 1850* (Harvard University Press, Cambridge, Mass., 1948, reprint), p.224.

4. L. Dock and M. Stewart, *A short history of nursing from earliest times to the present day* (Putnam, New York, 1920), p.154.

5. The first year of the Boston Training School for Nurses was considered to be unsuccessful. Although urged to give up the experiment, 'the trustees agreed to give the school another year of life provided a graduate nurse was placed in charge. The Committee procured Miss Linda Richards, a graduate of the New England Hospital for Women and Children, who had a year's experience during the formative period of the Bellevue.' The school was a success, and in 1896, was renamed the Massachusetts General Hospital Training School for Nurses.

6. *Massachusetts General Hospital memorial and historical volume together with the proceedings of the centennial of the opening of the*

hospital (Massachusetts General Hospital Reports, Boston, 1921), p.125.

7. Ibid., pp.52–127.

8. *Sixty-fifth Annual Report of the Superintendent of the McLean Asylum for the Insane to the Trustees of the Massachusetts General Hospital for the year 1882* (Massachusetts General Hospital Reports, Boston, 1882); Sixty-ninth Annual Report of the Trustees of the Massachusetts General Hospital and the McLean Asylum (Massachusetts General Hospital Reports, Boston, 1882).

9. E. Cowles, 'Nursing reform for the insane' *Am J. Insanity* (1904), p.176.

10. B. Chapin, *Am J. Insanity* (1904), p.116.

11. Ibid., p.176.

12. Ibid., p.178.

13. Ibid.

14. Ibid., p.182.

15. Ibid., p.183.

16. Ibid., p.184.

17. Ibid., p.186.

18. Ibid., p.187.

19. Ibid., p.191.

20. Ibid.

21. *Seventh Annual Report of the McLean Asylum Training School for Nurses* (Massachusetts General Hospital Reports, Boston, 1889), p.9.

22. Ibid., p.6.

23. J. S. and R. M. Haller, *The Physician and sexuality in Victorian America* (Norton, New York, 1978); H. R. Storer, *On nurses and nursing* (Lee and Shepard, Boston, Mass., 1868).

24. Storer, *On nurses and nursing*, p.16.

25. According to one account '. . . in order to become incorporated in 1901, it was necessary to ask the Canadians to withdraw'. In 1912, the organisation was renamed the National League of Nursing Education; S. E. Sly, 'A.N.A. growth since 1897' read before the fifteenth Annual Convention, Chicago, 5–7 June 1912.

26. M. E. May, 'Nursing of the insane' in I. A. Hampton *et al.*, *Nursing of the sick* (1893) (McGraw-Hill, New York, reprinted 1949).

27. I. A. Hampton *et al.*, *Nursing of the sick* (1893) (McGraw-Hill, New York, reprinted 1949), p.181.

28. J. B. Andrews, 'President's address before the American Medico-Psychological Association' *Trans. Am. Medico-Psychological Assoc.* (July 1893), p.52.

29. A. Clark, 'The future of asylum service'; C. B. Burr, 'What improvements have been wrought in the care of the insane by means of training schools?'; S. Smith, 'The proposed change of the legal status of the insane, in accordance with our present knowledge of the nature of insanity, for the purpose of securing for them more rational and efficient treatment.' *Am. J. Insanity* (1893–1894), p.50.

30. Proceedings of the American Medico-Psychological Association, Sixty-second Meeting, 12–15 June 1906 reprinted in *Trans. Am.*

Medico-Psychological Assoc., 13 (1906), p.203.

31. E. Cowles, *Trans. Am. Medico-Psychological Assoc.*, 13 (1906), p.203.

32. Ibid., p.204.

33. Ibid.

34. Ibid., p.206.

35. Ibid., p.207.

36. W. A. White, *Trans. Am. Medico-Psychological Assoc.*, 13 (1906), p.82.

37. *Report of the Committee on Training Schools for Nurses* American Medico-Psychological Association, 1907).

38. The Committee members were: George T. Tuttle, MD, Chairman; Charles P. Bancroft; Charles K. Clarke; Arthur W. Hurd; and William L. Russell. In their report they acknowledged the suggestions and criticisms provided by the following nurses: Miss Mary E. May, Willard State Hospital; Miss Marie Ferrier, Kings Park State Hospital; Miss Sara E. Parsons, Sheppard and Enoch Pratt Hospital; Miss Linda Richards, State Hospital for the Insane, Kalamazoo; and Miss Lucia E. Woodward, McLean Hospital.

39. *Report of the Committee on Training Schools for Nurses* (1907), p.3.

40. E. J. Taylor, 'Psychiatry and the nurse' *American Journal of Nursing*, 26(8) (1926), p.631.

41. E. J. Taylor, 'Nursing in the Henry Phipps Psychiatric Clinic' *Johns Hopkins Hospital Bulletin* (1915), p.26.

8

A History of the Visiting Nurse Association of Greater Kansas City: The First 75 Years

Laura Linebach

INTRODUCTION

The chilling wind nearly ripped Nurse Major's cloak out of her tightening grip. Carefully, she stepped off the front porch of the Morgan residence. Perhaps the Board of Managers of the Instructive Nursing Association could find someone to fix these loose boards. Certainly no one at this house could. While Mrs Morgan was pregnant with her seventh child, her husband had been killed at the packing house. Her oldest child was only eight, and he was too weak with pneumonia to even hold a hammer.

Nurse Major was a visiting nurse, the first visiting nurse in Kansas City, Missouri. She was tempted to dwell on all the problems of her last case, but there was not much daylight left and she must make two more visits before catching the street car back to the office to file her reports.

Pulling her cloak tightly around her and gripping her black bag of nursing equipment ever closer to her side, she marched down the street to the next case. 'In the next few months', Nurse Major thought, 'I will have an assistant, another graduate nurse. We need to reach more people and I can only go so far.'

Her feet were swollen by this time of day, but she barely noticed the pain for the cold February winds took away her breath. She concentrated on just breathing. That year, 1895, there had been so many ill, so many with fevers, consumption and pneumonia. She felt she could hardly feel sorry for herself when she saw with her own eyes the misery of so many in the town of Kansas City.

'Every city has its poor', she mused, thinking of her native England, where she had trained as a nurse. The whole idea of settlement and visiting nurses had begun in her homeland and, of course, Florence Nightingale was frequently consulted by nursing schools here in the States. Her own nursing association, which began in this booming town of Kansas City, was the third oldest in the States.

She reached the door of the next visit and knocked loudly. No one answered. 'That's strange', she thought. She knocked again and called, 'Mrs. Devlin!' Still no one answered. Her heart skipped a beat as she tried the door.

'Yes? Miss Major? Is that you?'

Nurse Major relaxed as she saw the steel blue eyes of Mrs Devlin.

'I was concerned you didn't answer, Mrs. Devlin.'

'I was almost too cold to get up and answer . . . until I thought it might be you. Do come in out of that dreadful wind.'

Nurse Major looked over her shoulder at the sun. She would have to be quick with this visit, even though lonely Mrs Devlin loved to chat with her about Ireland. She would just have to promise another visit soon. There were so many patients to visit, nurse, comfort, teach. So many . . .

THE VISITING NURSE ASSOCIATION OF GREATER KANSAS CITY

The evolution of the Visiting Nurse Association of Greater Kansas City followed the trend of other similar associations. In November 1889, the First Congregational Church Ladies' Union employed a trained nurse, Miss Lilly Major, to 'visit among the poor, without regard to color or denomination. A loan closet is kept, in which articles to be lent are given to the needy. Delicacies (food) are furnished, which are sometimes more useful than medicine.'[1] Just two years later the fledgling society met with its first financial difficulty.

In April 1891 . . . we find from the (church) annual report that several new plans of work announced at the last annual meeting had taxed the society to its utmost and that it had not been deemed advisable to enter upon any new work.[2]

So what was to become of the visiting nurse endeavour?

In October 1890, but for the timely assistance of the

gentlemen of the Church, the nursing work, an enterprise dear to the hearts of all, would necessarily have to be abandoned for lack of funds. They most generously responded to the appeal made to them and pledged a sufficient amount to carry it on until the first of May 1891, when it was thought a Nursing Association might be formed.[3]

An association would increase the scope of this work and thereby enable the union to better serve the community. A meeting of 'prominent women'[4] of Kansas City was called and there was no delay in forming the Instructive Nursing Association (INA). The objective of the Association was to:

Provide skilled nursing care to the sick in their home, to teach health and the prevention of disease. By means of cooperation with allied social agencies, assistance (was) rendered in the solution of social and economic as well as health problems.[5]

Mrs Henry Van Brunt was elected President, a position she held until 1900.

In 1890, there were approximately 21 visiting nurse associations in the United States and the idea spread even more rapidly after 1894. The Kansas City association is credited by one source with being the sixth oldest in the United States; another authority credits it with being the third oldest. The rankings vary due to the failure of other agencies or to the fact that others combined with existing visiting nurse associations.

The society page of the *Kansas City Times* (1892) gives a report of the first year's work of the INA

The first annual meeting of the Instructive Nursing Association was held in the Y.W.C.A. parlors, Wednesday forenoon, the President, Mrs. Van Brunt, in the chair . . . One trained nurse has been employed during the whole year and also emergency nurses when required. One hundred and forty-six have been cared for, 2,238 visits made by the nurses and 26 visits by members of the association. 202 articles have been loaned and 142 given from the linen closet. A number of pathetic cases were related of women and children suffering from illness aggravated by neglect, into whose lives a degree of order and comfort had been brought by . . . Miss Major, the nurse, whom one family has named 'Sunshine'. The Instructive feature of the work is always emphasised.[6]

Nurse Hill was added to the INA's staff in 1895. In 1897, another nurse, Miss Windicate, a recent graduate of the Scarritt School in Kansas City, applied to work for the Association. She desired to 'devote herself to work among the poor'.[7] However, since 'the City was in an apparently healthy condition' and a third nurse was not needed, she offered to volunteer her services during the vacation of Nurse Major and Nurse Hill. The Association was very particular about the nurses it hired. Applicants then, and for many years to come, went directly to the Board of Managers for approval. Board members were not afraid to express their doubts about certain applicants.

The Board cared a great deal for the INA nurses and worked with them on the smallest detail in order to run the Association effectively and professionally. They respected the nurses, particularly Nurse Major. The nurses were selected carefully, particularly since there was no state board criteria at the time. Requests presented at board of managers meeting on behalf of a nurse or client were rarely refused.

The Board of Managers met monthly and published reports to its members annually. Each Board member actively participated in the organisation through one of the various committees that had been formed. The Visiting Committee, for example, was set up to visit indigents and institutions. The Pay Committee reported the number of for-pay patient visits and amounts received and turned over to the Finance Committee. That Committee in turn made its report on the amount received from subscribers, membership fees and 'boxes'. These boxes were the collection boxes located throughout the city to receive donations for the INA. The Supplies Committee acknowledged gifts from members and other contributors; the Diet Committee had a budget used by Nurse Major to obtain fresh food.

When the Association left the umbrella of the First Congregational Church, it became incorporated and was very much on its own to raise the money needed to keep its work going. In the 1890s, occasional fund raisers were held. A vaudeville entertainment show in July of 1897 raised $127.20. Later that year, a diamond jubilee (for the Queen of England) fund-raiser netted the organisation a small amount of money. Photographs of the Queen's jubilee celebration were donated to the Visiting Nurse

Association (VNA) and were sold for a nickel each, yielding about $2.50.

The Association's first ten years — from the time the Ladies' Union first hired a trained nurse to the close of the century when that same nurse often required the assistance of other trained nurses — had been successful. A fledgling organisation operated by women who had not yet received the right to vote, was progressing well.

The start of the twentieth century saw social concern which was aimed at the institutionalised sick individual, with many local ordinances enacted to provide for hospitals and nurses to staff them.[8] While the Jackson County Medical Society pleaded for better city health measures, ordinances and commissions, the VNA became a powerful force in teaching health care to the poorest of the poor. The VNA was determined that these individuals not be lost in the midst of the smoke stacks of city progress.

In February 1900, 'the question came up as to the advisability of seeking paying patients when we have but one nurse as it is a charitable association, and at present as much as one nurse can do. If there is any time outside of the charity work, the nurse will be allowed to go.'[9] By this time, Mrs Givens, another nurse, assisted Nurse Major. She had begun her visits the previous year when Nurse Major was on vacation, and her services were used on a demand basis, as, for example, in March 1900 when several pneumonia cases had to be visited.

In late 1900, Nurse Major suffered 'an accident to her finger' and was 'unable to attend to her duties'. The benevolent Board agreed 'to pay Nurse Major her regular salary and $6.70 besides, which amount was used by Mrs Givens in car fares. Out of the regular salary, Mrs Givens was to have the amount agreed upon by the Board, which was set at a rate of $40 per month.'[10] This early account of 'workmen's compensation' was replicated in 1904, under similar circumstances; on that occasion, however, Nurse Major requested the Board turn over her salary directly to Mrs Givens 'so that double expense shall not be borne by the Association'.[11]

In 1904 patients were referred to the VNA by: previous patients (92); Provident Association (75); city physicians (26); other physicians (23); members of the Association (11); and miscellaneous sources (35). By 1909, these statistics changed considerably. Two hundred and twenty-three patients were referred that year by the Provident Association; one hundred and thirty-three by members; with seventeen coming from city physicians; seventeen from other physicians and one hundred and nineteen from other sources. The work grew considerably over the next five years, but for-pay patients (who had yielded $24.50 in 1904) provided only $63.20 in 1909.

The nursing staff was increased in 1904. Mrs Givens, originally hired to assist Nurse Major in emergencies, began seeing patients of her own. A nursing student, Miss Glazer of Scarritt Hospital, made eight visits that year as part of her training. Periodically, student nurses obtained public health training from VNA nurses. Also in 1904, the VNA divided Kansas City into districts for the delegation of work responsibilities.

The resignation of Nurse Major was announced on 6 December 1905. It was shocking news to the Board; meeting minutes stated 'The resignation of Miss Major was then presented to the Board who with much regret accepted it, but expressed the hope that after a year's rest . . . she might find herself able to take up the work once more.'[12] She had been with the VNA since its inception. For 16 years her work as a nurse had been invaluable in gaining the reputation that the Association needed to survive. She agreed to stay on until a suitable replacement was found. The following February, the Board decided to hire Mena Shipley, who had been active in the newly-formed Missouri Staff Nurses' Association and who had been appointed Chairperson of the Association's first Nominating Committee. In 1906, she in turn was replaced by a Miss Abshire.

A new plan was put into effect allowing patients to 'pay a small sum whenever able to do so to cover the car fare of the nurse thus helping our charity patients to help themselves and preserve their self-respect. This plan has been most successful in the Chicago Association and those of various eastern cities.'[13]

The Board members had taken personal interest and time to provide the nurses with distinguished, easily identified uniforms. A new badge was provided with the name of 'Visiting Nurse Association' rather than 'City Nurse'. 'This badge and a nurse in full uniform will be photographed, in order that the Metropolitan Company officers may recognise and pass our nurses freely . . .'[14]

The matter of proper uniform was finally settled on 6 March 1907. The Committee decided upon blue coat and bonnet. However, 'Miss Abshire refused to wear the bonnet and in consequence her resignation was requested to take effect on 15 March. The other nurses expressed their willingness to wear the becoming costume ordered.'[15] The uniform, readily identifiable, satisfied the transportation company and it agreed to allow VNA nurses to ride at no charge.

1907 was also the year when 'war was declared' on tuberculosis. The number of TB cases referred to the VNA rose over 400 per cent in one year — from 27 in 1907 to 110 in both 1908 and 1909. The $500 proceeds from a hospital dance association fundraiser was earmarked for the work. Mena Shipley, who had returned in 1909 to be Superintendent of the VNA, stated 'Since June, the services of one nurse has been almost entirely devoted to tuberculosis work, and her work has done little toward helping to stamp out the dread White Plague.'[16]

The Jackson County Society for the Relief and Prevention of Tuberculosis asked for the VNA's help in a sale of Red Cross stamps during that year's holidays; this was regarded by Miss Shipley as a sign of the recognition of the VNA's role in the fight against TB. By 1909 it appeared that:

> The people of Kansas City are slowly awakening to the fact that our Association is filling a great need, and that we are a help in many ways besides 'just caring for the sick.'[17]

Not only had the city noticed the existence of the VNA, but it was also co-operating in many ways. As the 1909 Annual Report noted, the Association was beginning a growth spurt.

Tuberculosis and maternal/child health became a worldwide concern, as it had been recognised by the Kansas City Visiting Nurse Association and various other health organisations. From 1910 to 1919 much of the growth of the VNA was due to first, recognition of the immense value of the visiting nurse for nursing health care and the patient teaching; and secondly, the co-operation of health organisations who wanted to expand services to their clients.

The first major corporation to recognise the value of the visiting nurse was the Metropolitan Life Assurance Company. Mena Shipley, VNA Superintendent, described the work extensively in the 1910 Annual Report. She wrote that the VNA service was not intended for those able to pay for large insurance but for those of small means.

It is bringing us in touch with a class of people we are anxious to reach — the self-respecting small wage earner . . . This service is absolutely free to policy holders. The service of one nurse is devoted entirely to Metropolitan Life Insurance work.[18]

Tuberculosis continued to receive considerable attention. In 1915, with the co-operation of the Jackson County Anti-Tuberculosis Society, the work was extended beyond the nurse, milk and eggs to the 'inauguration of the Open-Air School'. A VNA nurse was employed there for half a day each day caring for the needs of the children, under medical supervision.[19] In 1911, the VNA's work was again extended. In co-operation with St Luke's Hospital Club, the first baby day camps were established in the congested North End district and West Side. The babies were kept during the day and sent home at night during the months of July and August. This camp brought 'comfort and relief to so many sufferers during the unusually hot months of this last summer'.[20] Child care had thus become a major area of work to be handled by the VNA and was paid for by outside organisations.

The Red Cross Society established the Rural Nursing Service in 1912 to cover areas not included in the VNA's territory. In 1913, Miss Barr reported the significance of this work to the VNA:

The plan includes affiliation with already established visiting nurse associations as training fields for nurses who are to do rural work, and present staff opportunities for their local associations.[21]

Child welfare work extended to the Mattie Rhodes Day Nursery, where each week a nurse was sent to give practical demonstrations of the 'harmless but efficacious use of soap and water'. Mothers who had to leave their children while they went out to work could now be reassured that the children were well cared for and were being taught basic personal hygiene.[22]

The war years also had their effect on the VNA. Several nurses soon enrolled with the Red Cross and more followed later. But other events also had their impact on the VNA and its work at this time. The work for the Metropolitan Life Insurance Company on the Kansas side was transferred in June 1917 to the

Kansas City, Kansas, VNA. With the closure of the public schools also in June, one nurse was released from her work, while the Western Union took on its own nurse to care for its employees, 'making further visits by our nurses to the homes of employees unnecessary'.[23]

By the end of 1919, the nursing staff consisted of 26 nurses, most of whom were sponsored by philanthropic organisations. Much of the work was still supported by private contributions, memberships (life membership remained at $3 although most people gave more), bequests, endowments, fund-raisers and local charities. Following revision of the VNA's constitution, the Board applied for and received state charter, becoming an incorporated body, 'The Visiting Nurse Association of Kansas City, Missouri'.

Public health nursing continued to grow in importance across the country. By 1922 there were 15 postgraduate schools of public health nursing and 1800 nurses in that speciality. In 1926, that number had risen to 12,000. A frontier nursing service had been started in the rural areas of Kentucky in 1925, the nurses being known as 'the nurses on horseback', and the Indian Affairs Nursing Service had been operating for some time before.

In 1922 the Jackson County Medical Society approved a scheme for co-operating with the VNA to allow its nurses to make home visits for the Society. That same year, the two bodies co-operated further in a survey within Kansas City which identified and offered help to 'critically ill and crippled indigent children who were not receiving care or treatment . . . (VNA) nurses made 443 visits to these patients and a report of each case was sent from our office to the Jackson County Medical Society'.[24] Two further schemes with which the VNA became involved were the Negro Baby Welfare Clinic, opened in July 1922, and the work of an infantile paralysis clinic under the auspices of a special VNA committee, which began work in 1925.

Despite the obvious need for their services and the extending role which the VNA played in the health care of Kansas City, the VNA began losing nurses at the end of the 1920s. In part this was because of low pay; despite offering consistent raises, the pay which the VNA offered was not what nurses could earn elsewhere. The end of the decade saw a marked change in the fortunes of the VNA, with consequent effect on the pay rises it was capable of offering. At the beginning of 1928, the VNA had an operating balance of $5,859.40; by the end of 1929, that had become a deficit of $1,071.76. The 1930s were financially very difficult for the Association which struggled to keep its nurses in the clinics and in the homes.

Five nurses joined the VNA staff in June 1930, but by November the trend was toward a staff reduction. The Board looked for ways of overcoming the difficulties and still maintaining its range of services. It considered hiring practical nurses to 'visit patients only needing such service'. Student nurses were also seen as a way to save money, as often 'one of these students after graduation is employed on our staff and it saves much time otherwise lost in breaking in'.[25] The deficit continued, however, caused by failure to increase income, fewer paying patients and no increase in the number of insurance patients. People were unable to continue their insurance during the Depression years.

In an attempt to maintain the work level and service territory in the midst of a continual deficit budget, the VNA was asked to consider providing generalised — instead of specialised — nursing. The American Public Health Association argued that this would avoid duplication, lessen expenses and be more efficient. The Board voted unanimously to begin generalised nursing in the West Side District. Five nurses were assigned there in January 1931, with their headquarters at the Richard Cabot Club. These extra nurses were assigned to the infantile paralysis staff and, in the beginning, the transferring of records actually made their work harder. However, progress was made albeit slowly, and in May 1931 the South District was changed to generalised nursing except for TB work. In November that year, the East Side was also 'generalised'.

The beginning of 1937 painted a bleak picture for the Board. The staff had been reduced, by one means or another, from 61 in 1930 to 52. The salary cuts introduced in 1932 as a way of tiding the Association over the financial difficulties of the Depression had not been restored. Infantile paralysis work was increasing, and staff resignations and staff illness were all adding to the burden. In March that year, the new Social Security Act — which provided among other things for old-age benefits and unemployed insurance — came into force and it too proved to be an added financial burden for the Board.

How did the VNA manage to survive these financially trying times and still maintain its level of services to the poor? It was the determination of the Board not to cut services; the dedication of

133

those nurses who stayed not to cut quality nursing care; and the devotion of the community not to let the service of the VNA be lost at a time when it was most needed. However, if surviving the 1930s had been difficult, surviving the 1940s was to be even more so; it would be critical to the very existence of the VNA.

THE VNA IN THE 1940S

The Visiting Nurses Association had always prized its nurses, recognising that without them there could be no VNA. The nurses were held in esteem as individuals, uniquely qualified to make nursing judgements and thus provide the best care to those who trusted the VNA name. Like all Americans who had done their part sacrificing at home during the war, the VNA had its share of difficulties. The organisation was barely recovering from the Depression when the Second World War presented some even greater challenges.

In 1940, the budget deficit of $5,543.56 had risen to $6,217.18. About 91 per cent of the entire expenditure of the Association was for salaries, car fares and nursing supplies. There was no way of further reducing expenses without directly effecting the efficiency of the service provided. A survey in 1938 had recommended increasing the numbers of nurses, supervisors and clerical staff as well as salaries, but this was impossible to do. The staff was actually down from 61 in 1931 when generalised nursing had begun, to 49 in 1941. The limitations of staff and decrease in income placed a hardship on the remaining nurses. They were told to space visits farther apart and make 'fewer visits per case whenever possible in order to answer all the calls'.[26]

With America now fully involved in the war, ten VNA nurses volunteered in 1942 for the Army and two for the Navy. There were a total of eighteen resignations that year, with four vacancies at the end of the year. 'This turnover has been the greatest in more than twenty years and amounts to approximately 46% of the entire staff.'[27] The nurses had made a total of 80,104 visits to 15,554 patients in 1942, a loss of 12,144 visits and 4431 patients over the previous year. One reason for the drop in patients was the increasing number of people who, with hospitalisation insurance, chose to go into hospital for treatment rather than be cared for at home. A rise in average incomes among many of the former 'indigent' families took them out of the free care service but most were reluctant to pay for attention by the nurses of the VNA. The same applied to those mothers who had formerly used the free child health centres; better off, they were ineligible for free care but not so well off as to be able to take their babies to private physicians. Twenty-eight prenatal classes were begun and the VNA co-operated with the City Welfare Department in the matter of nursing service in nursery schools and day nurseries, services which 'increased in numbers due to war conditions'.[29]

In 1944, the VNA began accepting senior cadet nurses for a period of four to six months, a service offered to those who were interested in public health nursing and who were expected to engage in that branch of nursing after their training or military service. Despite the money which was saved by not replacing nurses when they left, the VNA was still in financial crisis. And of those nurses who left to take part in the war effort, few returned to the Association; many gave up work all together or had completely changed jobs. The Cadet Corps programme did not make up the deficit as had been hoped. The VNA was to be plagued by the shortage of nurses for many more years.

The VNA nurses now had a pension plan but their salaries remained below the minimum recommended by the National Organisation of Public Health Nursing. VNA staff nurses received a maximum of $180 for those without academic preparation and $190 for those with at least one year university work. The recommended scales were $200–$220 per month for nurses without academic preparation, and $210–$275 for those who had completed the approved one year programme of study in public health nursing. In 1946, the nurses were awarded a reduced working week; the 40-hour, 5-day working week was introduced with no loss in the number of visits nor service to patients. That was made possible by staggering the days off and ensuring that no district was left uncovered at any time. The number of student nurses at the VNA dropped dramatically that year, to only eleven for a full two-month affiliation. The sponsoring hospitals argued that they were unable to spare their students in the light of the shortage of nurses which they too experienced.[30]

By 1949, the VNA staff had diminished to twenty-nine including one physical therapist and the possibility of once again employing practical nurses to help out was considered. However, the Committee once again decided to delay introducing that measure. That decade ended on a very low note with the members of the Board being asked to carefully re-evaluate the whole VNA programme in the light of the financial and staff crises.[31]

THE VNA IN THE 1950S

The VNA was founded on the principle of the right of all individuals to health care. The task of bringing this care to the bedridden was basic to its incorporation. The cost challenges of maintaining the staff to serve so many were the problems which the VNA struggled with throughout the 1950s. The loss of staff, which had been going on for so many years, was not so great as the announcement made by the Metropolitan Life Insurance Company that it would discontinue its visiting nursing service to policy holders as of 1 January 1953. The decision represented an approximate loss of $5,000 per year to a budget already strained by a reduced contribution from the Community Chest Fund. In February 1950, the cost per visit increased from $2 per hour to $2.50, with $0.50 for each additional quarter hour. A charge of $1.50 was made for visits requiring a half-hour or less, such as those for administering hypodermics and changing dressings.

The loss of the Metropolitan Life contract was compounded by speculation that Blue Cross might also reduce the income available to the Association. But the doctors were also considered part responsible for the problems faced by the VNA. The VNA received 'surprisingly few referrals from doctors' in the Jackson County Medical Society but this was not so surprising.

> Suppose the patient needs three shots of penicillin. The doctor makes three house calls at $5 to $7.50 each, an income which he would be loathe to release. Yet the patient can have the visiting nurse for $1.50 per call, plus the cost of the penicillin. In this way, we become the doctor's competitor which understandably explains our small number of referrals from the . . . Society except in the case of non-paying patients.[32]

However, a public relations programme in 1952 did bring in more referrals during the next year from local physicians, which helped to make up the loss of income from the insurance companies. That same year, the VNA hired its first practical nurse, Mrs Dixon, a plan it had several times before rejected. Mrs Dixon was graduate of the School for Practical Nurses sponsored by the Vocational School of the Kansas City Board of Education. The VNA Board had decided at last that, as the training of the practical nurses was now being carried out in hospitals and not in placements to such organisations as the VNA, they would have to hire their own practical nurses.[33]

In 1955, the staff shortages were once again felt deeply. The previous year two nurses had resigned within a week of their appointment because 'the work was too hard'.[34] The budget allowed for a staff of twenty-nine, but there were only one director, four supervisors, nineteen registered graduate nurses, one practical nurse and two clerical personnel on the staff in 1955. Fewer visits were made that year, but as the executive director, Audrey Holt remarked about the statistics, 'Quality of service can never be measured by numbers.'[35] The following year she returned to that theme:

> We cannot take credit for making more visits in 1956 than in 1955 but we do hope we have made better visits. No two visits are the same. Just as each patient is a different individual, even though his illness may be the same as his neighbor's, the nursing care he receives is built around his own personal need.[36]

In 1960, the VNA filled all staff positions provided for in the budget. Nurses continued to receive extra training in order to be registered nurse-physical therapists. Nursing care visits were $3 for any period up to an hour and $0.50 for each additional quarter hour. Nurse-therapists' calls were $3.50 and $0.50 respectively. The maximum salary for a staff nurse was increased to $350 per month and the total estimated expenditure of the association for 1960–1 was $139,426 of which $116,840 came from the Community Chest. With this more encouraging picture in mind, the VNA prepared once more for expansion, as the city grew apace in the 1960s.

In response to that expansion and the need for tighter financial control, the Association adopted a statistical method of reporting nursing activities, beginning in October 1962. 'One big change is that we count an individual only once on any particular service — whereas in the past they could be dismissed and reopened in the year and recounted.'[37] There were also problems

137

in recovering payments for visits, particularly from the 'indigents' who received public assistance.

In 1965, two doctors on the staff at the General Hospital asked the VNA to participate in a new treatment regime for emphysema. The Board agreed and one VNA staff nurse of the time recalled the programme as significant because it was a time when nursing began to branch out into more sophisticated care in the home, and moved away from doing baths and giving injections and routine treatments. The same year, a visiting health aide programme was looked at. A pilot scheme started in late 1965 to last until July 1966, when it was evaluated. Health aides were expected to carry out functions which could be performed by a knowledgeable family member if one were available. They worked under the supervision of the VNA registered nurse.

Medicare was passed on 20 July 1965 and became effective on 1 July 1966. According to an article in the *Kansas City Times*, a survey of local population at the time (79,000 persons 65 and older) showed that 5000 Kansas citizens would need recurrent home care. But the VNA had already cared for 6709 persons in this age group the previous year. The VNA estimated that at least 59 nurses would be required to meet this demand; at that moment, there were just 38 on staff.

An early discharge programme was also introduced in 1966 and 1967 through links between the VNA and local hospitals. The programme reduced health care costs to the patient, freed scarce hospital beds for the more seriously ill and helped speed up the recovery of discharged patients.[38] A medical social worker was added to the VNA staff in 1968 to co-ordinate efforts to find additional community resources for VNA patients. According to one of the VNA directors, Helen C. Green, VNA nurses learnt how to separate public health nursing from social work by combining the expertise of two professionals to produce results and action.[39]

The 1960s then, ended on a high note with the Association once more in an expansive and innovative mood. The challenges remained but so did the excitement of facing them. In her executive director's report of 1968–9, Helen Green wrote:

My emphasis today is to look forward to next year and the coming years. Will we be able to continue to grow? — not with emphasis on size but in depth of program — quality care, improved case finding to reach those in need of nursing care, continuity of care through coordinated programs, prevention of fragmentation through health planning for the Greater Kansas City area.[40]

CONCLUDING REMARKS

Health care in the 1970s, with its rising prices and government intervention on Medicare and Medicaid controls, began to demand more and more consumer input as well as nursing input. Health care was seen by the end of the 1970s as belonging to all, as a right — not a privilege — even without a national health insurance plan. The VNA, characteristically, had always taken that view, never turning away patients because of low income.

In the 1970s, the VNA grew concerned that people were not being appropriately referred for home health care after discharge following hospitalisation. It appointed a co-ordinator of hospitals, Bernadina Knipp, RN, and community care was assured because 'time is not lost, nor does regression occur before home care is given'.[41] A hospital co-ordinator group, representing the different hospitals in the area, met to share information about patient dismissal planning, available resources, problems encountered and ways to overcome these.

The year 1971 brought financial difficulties to the VNA once again. Increased costs, decreasing Medicare payment and a failure to get an increase in grant were responsible. But despite this, the VNA continued to extend and innovate.

A speech therapist was added to the staff in 1971. The health aide programme was expanded and the total staff now resembled the services provided by hospitals. 'We care for sicker patients discharged earlier from hospital or perhaps not even in the hospital. Their problems are complex', explained Helen Green. Later, in 1978, a dietitian was appointed to participate in team meetings, act as consultant with staff and provide instruction to clients at nutrition sites.

Home health care once again became the focus of attention in the 1980s as home health agencies began springing up almost overnight. Patients were receiving more and more treatments in the home, shortening their hospital stays and saving money for themselves and insurance companies alike. The VNA entered the 1980s with renewed optimism that home health care was reaching heights never before dreamed of by its founders in the

1890s. To meet this new challenge, a mission statement (Appendix 1) was drawn up in June 1980 which defined the present and future goals of the agency and a three-year plan was adopted to meet the objectives set by the mission statement. By 1981, the VNA had grown to a team of 216 nurses, service providers, administrative and office support staff. By 1982, this number increased to 240. Included in these totals were now a mental health specialist and an oncology specialist.

The history of the Visiting Nurse Association Home Health Services of Greater Kansas City was replicated across the United States. From its origins as a small-scale philanthropic religious endeavour to a complex community-based health care programme, the VNA consistently sought to serve the needs of the poor and the sick. The financial insecurity which marked its early years — the struggle for bequests; subscriptions and fund-raisers — were echoed and exacerbated in the middle decades of the twentieth century. Two features mark out the VNA. First, its commitment to care in the home for the poor and the sick on the basis of need rather than ability to pay and on the basis of individuality. Second, the development of nursing practice largely uninhibited by medical politics and ideology. The nursing model may well be of contemporary debate: it was, nevertheless, constructed, evaluated, extended and practised by the home nurses of the Greater Kansas City Visiting Nurse Association.

NOTES

1. B. B. Leelye, *A brief history of the Congregational Church* (Hailman Co., Kansas City, 1909), p.48.
2. Ibid., p.49.
3. Ibid.
4. *History: 50 years of visiting nurse service* (VNA of Kansas City, Mo., Kansas City, 1939).
5. Edwin A. Christ, *Missouri's nurses* (E.W. Stevens, Columbia, 1957), p.266.
6. *Kansas City Times* (10 April 1892).
7. Minutes, Board of Managers, Visiting Nurse Association (VNA minutes) (2 June 1897), p.8.
8. Christ, *Missouri's nurses*, pp.92–4.
9. VNA minutes (7 February 1900), p.76.
10. VNA minutes (2 January 1901), p.92.
11. VNA minutes (7 December 1904), p.27.
12. VNA minutes (6 December 1905).
13. Annual Report, Visiting Nurse Association (VNA Annual

Report) (1 January 1906–31 December 1906), pp.5–6,8.

14. VNA minutes (6 February 1907), p.85.

15. VNA minutes (6 March 1907), pp.87–8.

16. VNA Annual Report (1 January 1909–31 December 1909), p.9.

17. Ibid.

18. VNA Annual Report (1 January 1910–1 January 1911), pp.10–11.

19. VNA Annual Report (1 January 1915–1 January 1916), p.4.

20. VNA Annual Report (1 January 1911–1 January 1912), p.5.

21. VNA Annual Report (1 January 1913–1 January 1914), p.8.

22. VNA Annual Report (1 January 1914–1 January 1915), p.1.

23. VNA Annual Report (1 January 1917–1 January 1918), p.9.

24. VNA Annual Report (1 January 1923), p.10.

25. Minutes, Board of Trustees, Visiting Nurse Association (VNA Trustees Minutes) (11 June 1930)

26. Director's report (Director's report) for the year ending 31 December 1941, p.1.

27. Director's report (1942).

28. Ibid., pp.1–2.

29. VNA Trustees minutes (9 December 1942).

30. Director's report (1946), p.1.

31. President's report (President's report) for the year ending 31 December 1949, p.2.

32. President's report (1952), p.2

33. Director's report (1953), p.1.

34. Director's report (1954), pp.4–5.

35. Director's report (1955), p.4

36. Director's report (1956), p.7.

37. Director's report (1963), p.3.

38. Director's report (1967), p.1.

39. Director's report (1969), p.2.

40. Ibid.

41. Report to the Board of Trustees of the Visiting Nurse Association of Greater Kansas City, Mo. (11 February 1970).

APPENDIX 1

The VNA Mission Statement

The mission of the Visiting Nurse Association Home Health Services of Greater Kansas City is:

to offer community-based home health care and related services to the people of Greater Kansas City and neighbouring areas;

141

to provide high quality home health care and related services in a cost-effective manner;

to provide services which are preventive, treatment orientated, educational and rehabiliative in nature;

to utilise available resources in its approach to patient care and direct services appropriate to the needs of the individual;

to meet community needs for home health care and related services through utilisation and co-ordination of regional and local planning efforts, other health care providers and the medical community as resources in determining and serving those needs;

to expand its service area and the scope of services offered to the extent these services meet a need and can be provided with quality and cost-effectiveness to the patient;

to take a position of leadership in educating health care professionals and the public in home health care; and

to set a standard of excellence for home health care and related services in the areas it serves.

9

For the Good of the Patient?

Ruth Hawker

INTRODUCTION

Local historical studies can both complement and challenge macro-historical accounts. This is particularly evident in the history of nursing where national studies have frequently failed to take note of regional and local differences in development. There are many documents relevant to the local situation held in public record offices or hospital archives which have seldom been consulted. They vary in quantity and quality from area to area, but once located can provide a rich source of data that can either support identified trends or generate further questions about a specific local or national issue.

In this chapter some of the issues raised by the notion 'for the good of the patient' will be discussed using primary source documents from the eighteenth and nineteenth centuries relating to the organisation of one provincial hospital, the Royal Devon and Exeter Hospital, located in South-West England and founded in 1743. This present work has been stimulated by evidence which came to light while working on another major study.[1] In the course of the research for that study, two letters, which will be discussed in detail later in this chapter, came to light which suggested that a proposed organisational change was justified because it would be in the 'best interests of the patients'.

The discussion begins with a general description of what it was like to be a patient in the Royal Devon and Exeter Hospital (Exeter Hospital) during this early period. Some of the constraints on patient behaviour that were considered important by the hospital authorities and those who controlled the institution are discussed. There then follows an analysis of whether or not the events described can be said to have been primarily 'for the good of the patient'.

EXETER AND ITS PEOPLE

The inhabitants of Georgian Exeter have been described as 'wealthy, lively, bustling and as narrow as its streets in some respects'.[2] The commercial prosperity of the city, based on the then thriving wool trade, attracted merchants from many parts of England, as well as from Germany and Holland, to settle in the area. Each of these new households employed large numbers of servants, both indoor and outdoor, while the increase in the building industry also provided plenty of opportunities for the employment of artisans. This 'bustling' prosperity attracted many people into the city from the surrounding countryside.

It was in this affluent environment that Dean Alured Clarke, who had previously been actively involved in the establishment of the hospital at Winchester, appealed at the beginning of 1741 for monetary contributions in order to provide a service for the 'sick poor'. These individuals were those who did not have a family to provide for them in times of need. Indeed, many of these 'sick poor' were the employees of the wealthier Exeter citizens who were now asked to help establish a hospital to take care of them.

The interdependence of these two groups — the wealthy merchants and their employees, the 'sick poor' — was referred to during the ceremony to lay the foundation stone of the new hospital later that same year. It was reported that the Dean made:

> an excellent and solemn oration . . . offering up his prayers to the Almighty for success in the undertaking, recommending to those who were in affluent circumstances the duty of assisting the poor in times of sickness, and exhorting the poor to be obedient to their superiors, and grateful to their benefactors.[3]

THE HOSPITAL PATIENTS

The patients who were eventually admitted to the hospital

were expected to be duly grateful not only to their earthly benefactors but also to the Almighty. One of the hospital rules stipulated that before discharge, each patient should, in the presence of an officer of the hospital, offer up a prayer of thanksgiving for the help received. The rule continued to be enforced until at least 1912.[4] Obedience was enforced by the strict interpretation and application of a set of rules drawn up by the Board of Governors. If any rule was broken, the patient was immediately discharged and his or her name put on a 'black list' which was displayed on a wall in the ward as a warning to others. Once blacklisted, a patient could not return to the hospital 'on any pretence whatever'. A copy of the rules was hung in the ward and a Visitor was appointed by the Governors to inspect the hospital each week to ensure that the rules were not being broken.

The Visitor might be a member of the Board of Governors or one of the subscribers to the hospital, but was appointed specifically to the post by the Board. The Visitor also ensured that the staff obeyed the rules of the institution. A similar code of behaviour to that imposed on the patients applied to members of the staff, and the Governors were equally ruthless or strict with employees who transgressed. Instant dismissal was the automatic response to any infringement of the code of conduct.

The early patients were expected, also on pain of dismissal, to help with the domestic tasks of the institution. Children were required to fetch any potions used by the apothecary. Female patients were expected to carry and to serve food to those patients who were too ill to shift for themselves. Male patients had to help the staff pump the water from the hospital well and also tend the hospital pigs which were kept in the yard.

The threat of instant dismissal which applied to both patient and employee appears to have served the needs of the institution rather than the good of the patient. However, there are indications that at times the administrators could make decisions which could work for the good of the patient as well as the good of the organisation. For example, male patients had to help the staff draw water. This appears to have been an onerous task as well as an unpopular one, disliked by both staff and patients. The employees insisted that all male patients take their turn, unless so ill as to be incapable. The matter was obviously contentious and, during one dispute in 1793, was referred to the Governors for resolution. The Governors decided that all patients who were well enough had to carry out this task but that the doctor had first to decide whether an individual was fit enough to take part. Those whom the doctor decided were capable of helping to draw water were identified by a red P placed above their bed. The letter showed that they were considered well enough to be used in the domestic chores of the hospital including the dreaded pumping. However, this decision, enforced by the doctor's examination and 'certification', actually meant that the number of patients available to help with the domestic chores was considerably reduced.

RELATIVES AND FRIENDS AND PATIENTS

The hospital rules applied equally to the relatives of the inpatients. Visiting was allowed but relatives were forbidden to bring in any food or liquor. This rule was later amended, during the nineteenth century; all food continued to be forbidden, but it was now *expected* that tea and sugar would be supplied by the patient's relatives or friends. An appeal to the Governors by the family of a patient unable to supply these basic commodities met with a negative response. The Committee stated that these could not be provided by the hospital authorities 'on any account'; the decision and the rule change clearly related to the contemporary price of the two items as well as their popularity amongst the working classes.

The rule designed to prevent food being brought in for patients was difficult to enforce. The records for 1830 indicate that despite strict measures including searching relatives as they entered the hospital, and searching the patients' lockers after visiting time was over (a practice which continued well into the twentieth century), the practice continued. After this period of time, it may be difficult to understand why this particular rule was so strictly enforced by the Exeter Governors, particularly since the practice in other English hospitals was so different. For example, at Guy's Hospital, London, relatives were positively encouraged to provide food for the patients and food sellers, including a watercress seller, visited the wards to ply their wares.[5] One possible explanation for the breach of this rule may be because sharing food is a social act of some significance; the provision of food from home, particularly when home was in a rural setting like Exeter, surrounded by rich agricultural land, was seen by many patients as an important way of maintaining their links with their family and home.

The nursing staff of the Exeter Hospital had to search the lockers after visiting times. The medical staff were also involved in enforcing this particular rule. According to the newspaper report of an inquest held in 1889, it was stated in evidence by the mother of the deceased patient that:

> She knew he (the patient) had an appetite, but they would not allow him what he wanted. He did not say what he had been denied. He asked a witness to bring him in some sweets but the nurse said they were not allowed. A sponge cake or two had been taken to him, but he was not permitted to eat them.

In reply, the house surgeon in his evidence stated that 'The rules of the Institution did not permit such things being taken to the patient and he had to act almost as a detective at times to prevent things being smuggled in.'[6]

Other constraints were put on patients. Smoking was forbidden and also playing cards and other games of chance. Patients who could read were allowed to do so, but the reading material provided by the hospital was controlled from 1829 onwards by a group of five clergymen who were required to 'select such works upon a list of the Society for Promoting Christian Knowledge, as shall to them appear fit to be placed in the several wards for the use of the patients'.[7]

NURSING AT THE ROYAL DEVON AND EXETER

The routinisation of nursing care came about gradually during the latter half of the nineteenth century. Patients were initially expected to assist with the day to day domestic arrangements. Their daily activity during the first 60 years following the establishment of the hospital was inextricably bound up with that of the nurse. The first nurses appointed to the hospital were mostly drawn from the same social class as the patients. They were 'not above the ranks of those who became housekeepers and servants'.[8] Whilst some were dismissed for breaking the rules of the institution, most appear to have conformed to the discipline of the hospital and were kindly, well-meaning women. One consultant witnessed the hospital in the nineteenth century through its pre- and post nursing reform eras; he saw in the reformed nursing system the 'better class of nurse with more general information and power of perception', but he also had some regard for the old-style nurses. 'They had a homeliness about them that made the patients, especially the old folk, feel at home in the hospital . . . they could enter into the troubles of their patients and act as an intermediary.'[9]

The early nurses were well placed to 'enter into the troubles of their patients' for they shared accommodation by sleeping in a partitioned-off section of the ward. Patients and nurses also ate together in the ward; and shared the domestic chores between them. During the eighteenth century, the nurse certainly assisted the doctor but in a very limited way. She helped with dressings, but only by fetching tins of warm water for the doctor. She was allowed to apply bread or linseed poultices but the rule was that 'as soon as dressings of lotion and lint were ordered, the pupil will take charge'.[10] The pupils were young men who would eventually go on to complete some form of medical training, but who were employed as assistants to the doctors or the apothecary.

A redefinition of the role of both the nurse and the patient began around the 1830s. There was very little surgery carried out initially, apart from 'cutting of the stone' and few casualties were seen and admitted to the hospital. However, at the beginning of the nineteenth century the need for a casualty ward became apparent; the number of patients presenting after accidents on the many building sites in the city rose significantly. The amount of surgery carried out also increased and eventually the first 'operation nurse' was appointed in 1835.

At this time, balneo-therapeutics (warm baths) was fashionable for a wide range of ailments. The baths, which included hot, cold, sulphur and vapour baths, were administered jointly by the nurses and the pupils. They were probably the first procedure for which nurses were seen to be important.

Although patients and nurses continued to share some aspects of their life, the changing and extending role of the nurse may have both distanced her from the patient and had adverse effects on her charges. It was at this time that some patients appeared to be so dissatisfied with their conditions that the Governors were recording their anxiety that two or three patients were 'escaping' each week from the hospital.[11]

Relatives were also expressing their discontent at change and the restrictions put upon them by the Governors. Prior to one

Sunday visiting hour, 'a great tumult' formed outside the hospital which could not be controlled by the porter. The Governors appealed to the Mayor to help prevent future disturbances of that nature.

The pupil system gradually died out in the nineteenth century. In part, this was due to the replacement of the apothecaries by qualified doctors. The doctors also began to drop the apprenticeship system of employing young, unqualified men to gain experience before formal training in the medical schools. Consequently, the nurses carried out more and more of the duties hitherto performed by the pupils. In order to complete this increased work load, the patients' day was extended and work began much earlier.

Formal nurse training began in Exeter in 1888; however, before that date a new matron 'of the same educated type' had been appointed, and the local women who made up the bulk of the nursing staff were engaged 'under certain rules' and given some measure of training before appointment to the permanent staff of the hospital. As the 'new' sisters gradually replaced the existing members of the nursing staff, the routine of the patients' day became even more rigid — woken at 5.45 a.m. and lights out at 8 p.m. In addition to the rules of the institution, patients now had a strict regime with which to comply.

It was in the course of these dramatic changes in the latter half of the nineteenth century that the notion 'for the good of the patient' was first put forward. Both the matron and one of the doctors used the idea in an appeal to the Governors once again over control of the visiting arrangements. Numerous attempts had been tried to control visiting throughout the period.[12] In 1871, the newly appointed matron and the houseman expressed concern about the number of visitors allowed in to visit each patient at any one time. Both sent letters of complaint to the Governors and the hospital authorities. The house surgeon pointed out that because there was no limit to the number of visitors allowed, 'in consequence the wards are sometimes much too crowded *to the discomfort and injury to the sick*'. The matron asked the Governors to restrict the number allowed in and concluded her letter by stating that 'frequently one patient has seven visitors in three-quarters of an hour. *It does much harm to the patient*'[13] (emphasis added).

The Governors acquiesced and introduced a ticket system that continued until the 1950s. Only two people were allowed to have

149

a ticket and to visit at any one time. While this resolved the position in the wards to the satisfaction of the nurses and the doctors, it meant that, whatever the weather, other members of the family were forced to wait outside the hospital for the ticket holder to come out and hand over the ticket so that they might go in. It was not until 20 years later, in 1892, that the editor of one of the local newspapers drew his readers' attention to this. He argued that visitors who had become cold and perhaps wet from standing outside might not be the best visitors for the patients. The Governors relented in the face of this publicity and permitted visitors to wait in the outpatients' hall if the weather was inclement.[14]

An examination of local sources provides examples of the ways in which a Board of Governors of a hospital — and later the doctors and nurses as well — controlled patient behaviour. Towards the end of the nineteenth century such controls were said to be 'for the good of the patient'. That notion, which forms part of hospital life, has been described by Coser (1962)[15] as functional for the professional because it serves to strengthen common norms. Coser argues that the dividing line between 'for the good of the patient' and 'for the good of the organisation' (or professional) cannot easily be demonstrated. The patient thus becomes a 'disembodied abstraction'.

Contemporary studies of nursing and health care in this country also suggest that this disembodied abstraction appears to be a relatively unimportant part of the organisational structure of the hospital and that the present social structure mitigates against active involvement by the patient in decision making about his or her care.[16] Conformity of behaviour on the part of the patient and relative is still expected by hospital staff, and it has been shown that the nurse will adopt specific behaviour in order to produce that conformity.[17] As an example, in order to implement the rules and policy decisions relating to the control of visiting, the nurse has traditionally adopted the role of gatekeeper on behalf of the institution.

In this chapter we began by discussing the original aims of the organisation, the Royal Devon and Exeter Hospital. At first glance, it would appear that it was an institution specifically designed to meet the needs of the patient. If we take into account the wider social environment of Georgian and Victorian England, the rules of the hospital resemble many of the structures of contemporary society. It is therefore unsurprising that both staff and patients were expected to conform to the rules within the institution. But there is no doubt that the Governors saw in the rules the means for controlling an institution which might otherwise have been chaotic. The service they offered was conditional upon the patients' conformity. The patients were drawn almost exclusively from the employed classes; service to 'superiors' was expected and generally given. Those who failed to give that service did not remain in employment. The hospital also required that the patient be 'recommended' by a subscriber and this in turn encouraged conformity. However, the strict application of the rules of the hospital led to 15 per cent of all patients being discharged because they failed to accept the discipline. Staff were also dismissed without compensation for 'irregularity'. The needs of the institution, then, were paramount, despite those few occasions when the Governors appear to have acted in the interests of the patients.

Hospital life for the patient during the eighteenth century was similar to that for the nurse. Both had to submit to a rigidly disciplined regime, but because of their shared social status they had a common understanding which drew them together and apart from the institution. That shared experience disappeared with the introduction of the new nursing system after the mid-nineteenth century. The reforms introduced to 'improve' patient care may well have not been perceived as such by the recipients of that improved nursing care.

Much of the evidence available locally supports the notion that, in almost every instance, the interests of the patient were secondary to those of the institution or the professionals. The Governors exerted control over the organisation by a code of rules; this was enforced by the appointment of the Hospital Visitor; later control was exercised on behalf of the Governors by the nurses and doctors. The patients, with the exception of those who were dismissed or who 'escaped', played a very passive role in the process.

Social control is an important element in the structure of organisations. The legitimisation of control forms an important part of the process of professionalisation and nowhere is this more evident than in the history of nursing and of hospitals in the modern period. The focus on local issues highlighted in this paper helps illuminate that aspect of institutional life and demonstrates the need to pose the question, 'in whose interest is change sought?'

NOTES

1. R. J. Hawker, 'The interaction between nurses and patients's relatives', unpublished thesis, University of Exeter, 1982.

2. W. G. Hoskins, *Two thousand years in Exeter*, 2nd edn (Phillimore and Co., Chichester, 1963).

3. Hoskins, *Two thousand years in Exeter,* p.88.

4. Rules for ward sisters, Royal Devon and Exeter Hospital, 1912.

5. H.C. Cameron, *Mr. Guy's hospital 1726–1948* (Longman Green, London, 1954).

6. *Devon and Exeter Daily Gazette* (12 January 1889).

7. Minutes of the Central Committee, Royal Devon and Exeter Hospital, 1829.

8. J. Delpratt Harris, *The Royal Devon and Exeter Hospital* (Eland Bros., Exeter, 1922).

9. Ibid.

10. Ibid.

11. Minutes of the Central Committee, Royal Devon and Exeter Hospital, 1832.

12. R. J. Hawker, 'Rules to control visitors 1746–1900', *Nursing Times* (21 March 1984), pp.49–51.

13. Minutes of the Central Committee, Royal Devon and Exeter Hospital, 1871.

14. Minutes of the Central Committee, Royal Devon and Exeter Hospital, 1982.

15. R. L. Coser, *Life in the ward* (Michigan State University Press, East Lancing, Mich., 1962).

16. See for example, Alan Davis (ed.), *Relationships between doctors and patients* (Teackfield, Farnborough, 1978).

17. R. J.Hawker, 'Gatekeeping: a traditional and contemporary function of the nurse', in R. White (ed.), *Political issues in nursing: past, present and future* (John Wiley and Son, Chichester, 1985).

10

From Individual Dedication to Social Activism: Historical Development of Nursing Professionalism

Cynthia Q. Woods

Questions about whether nursing qualifies as a profession and the nature of nursing professionalism have been discussed in nursing literature since its earliest days. This chapter will trace the historical development of nursing ideology as reflected in the writings of nursing leaders and medical sociologists. It reveals the expansion of the conception of nursing professionalism from an internal quality, defined by personal values, to an attribute oriented to dynamic, external factors of practice as well.

Elliot Freidson, a leading medical sociologist, called health care the most professionalised of all human sciences, and said:

> What is special about professionals is believed to be a stable set of ethical and other kinds of values which guide their behavior . . . There is the assumption that attitudes and values — ethics and dedication — are more important than the circumstances in which they are tested. The assumption itself . . . is one espoused by the profession, which sees itself as a group with a special kind of knowledge and a special state of mind rather than a group organized in a special way.[1]

Freidson felt that this ideological individualism blocks a profession from understanding behaviour of its members, from understanding that structural characteristics of a profession have far more influence on the nature of care than good intentions and skills of individual members. This concept is as useful in understanding the successes and failures of attempts to promote professionalism in nursing as in medicine.[2]

In her recent text, Lucie Young Kelly described fairly general agreement that professionalism centres on specialised expertise, autonomy and service.[3] Bixler and Bixler's characteristics of a profession, modelled after Flexner's classic criteria, have achieved wide acceptance by many professionals. [4,5] Kelly maintained that, though there are weaknesses in nursing's achievement of criteria related to its body of knowledge, education in higher institutions and career orientation, the most serious weakness is lack of autonomy. Lewis and Batey defined autonomy as 'freedom to make discretionary and binding decisions consistent with one's scope of practice and freedom to act on those decisions'.[6] Recognition and discussion of these themes of structural relationships and autonomy gradually emerge in twentieth-century writings about nursing professionalism.

Professionalism has appeared as a topical heading since the earliest indices to nursing literature, but autonomy, power, politics and political action did not appear until the late 1960s. Though thinking on these topics and the interrelationship of the two aspects of professionalism, internal ideology and external organisation and structure of practice, can be surmised, it is rarely made explicit in early writings. Nursing practice surely mirrored the larger culture and social ideologies about women, education, health and professionalism. One wonders how accurately writing by nurses 'reflects their own behaviour and how much did they reflect ideology or wishful thinking? How close was their self-image to the reality of their daily care?'[7]

Florence Nightingale's insistence on structuring early schools of nursing independently from hospitals, with paid nurse instructors, seems to indicate her appreciation of the importance of autonomy. Nevertheless, she clearly relied on what Freidson called common-sense individualism to insure that graduate nurses would continue to perform in the desired manner, regardless of the setting or structure later imposed.

This view and her opposition to nurse registration are consistent with Freidson's analysis that:

> Our civilization emphasizes choice over constraint, the individual over the group, and the actor over the environment . . . Our instinct is to analyze the human world by reference to the individual motives, values and knowledge rather than by reference to the organization of the human world itself.

Freidson felt this orientation resulted in two assumptions. The first, seeing the world as made up of individuals, overlooks the constraints and limits that the social environment places on behaviour, regardless of personal qualities. The second assumption is that 'individual characteristics are definitely formed at some point of time into a stable and fixed bundle of knowledge, motives and values and that therefore he will act . . . more or less the same way no matter the environment he acts in may be'.[8]

Both of these assumptions are implicit in the movements for registration and formal education of nurses as a means to professionalisation. Gradually nursing leadership came to see these means as necessary but not sufficient to realise the goal of professional autonomy.

The spirit of reform and the nationally popular progressive ideology that brought the food and drug administration, the public health movement and the reform and regulation of medicine obviously influenced nursing leaders. In 1902 Linda Richards proudly wrote of a number of nurses providing leadership in health related civic and community activities such as settlement work and even the study of law, sociology and modern movements.[9]

The drive for licensure or registration in Great Britain and the US at the turn of the century was the first political effort of a large number of nurses concerned with establishing control of the evolving profession. Within eight years, 1903 through 1911, thirty states adopted nurse registration laws.[10] Lavinia Dock also advanced concerns for nursing and women's issues such as suffrage and venereal disease and chastised nursing organisations for not becoming more involved.[11]

Dock seemed more sensitive than most to the often unrecognised importance of the work setting and political power. And yet she presented a touchingly naive blend of idealism and wishful thinking about nursing with her fervent plea that nurses support the union movement for shorter hours for *other* hospital workers and better wages for *teachers*. As for nurses, she said:

Eager to throw ourselves into the crises of our own tasks, which are indescribably dramatic because they hinge always on the acutest questions of life and death, we have resented any interference with hours of work and have echoed the sentiment too often skillfully suggested by hospital directors personally interested, that a 'profession' must become tainted with 'trades unionism' and that legal ordering of working hours would . . . destroy professional ethics.[12]

Was she expressing naivete or sarcasm?

Though the following quotation seems to reflect less dominance of nursing by medicine than later on, Dock seemed to foresee the trap of professional narrowness and inertia that plagued nursing for so long when she wrote:

> We and our professional brothers, the doctors, have fallen into a way of assuming superiority and aloofness . . . if we are exclusive and shut our minds to all except 'professional' subjects we shall become one sided specialists and in time lose our usefulness.[13]

Was nursing a profession? One of the earliest writings on the subject was by a physician. A supporter of nursing education, he said 'The profession of nursing, like that of medicine, is an art dependent on science, but in nursing, important as is the underlying science, the art must always predominate.'[14] He nevertheless expressed the common doubts about the wisdom or possibility of a scientific knowledge base for nursing. Despite the sexist touch of crediting Theodor Fliedner as the rightly called father of nursing, Worcester said modern nursing met his five tests of a profession: (1) teaching their successors, (2) sharing professional advantage and making their own professional regulations, (3) acknowledging the need for continuous study, (4) pursuing their profession not primarily for pecuniary gain, and (5) requiring sufficient education of those who enter the profession. Finally, he implied recognition of the constraints of practice organisation and setting, contributing to the 'sometimes unprofessional conduct' of private nurses and to the upholding of the highest standards by district nurses.

The 1920s brought extension and consolidation of the power and prestige of medicine and the superior/subordinate relationship of medicine and nursing. And the relationship between the two disciplines has continued to be a powerful determinant of nursing's development.

At the inception of organized nursing, nurses in many ways were the equals of physicians in their professional training and their contributions to the health care of society. However, they were not their equals in the political and economic spheres of human activity, or in influence on the public, and it was this lack of equality that would shape their development far more than their professional ideals.[15]

The stereotype of women as unscientific and saintly long remained part of nursing's professional image. Graciously appreciative though he was of 'refined and well-educated young women who tend the sick', Dr Cabot, of Boston, assured his audience in 1923 that nurses sought such work:

> not primarily to earn a living or to contribute to science. Of course they want some money as a result, but they don't enjoy the process or seek money for its own sake . . . In the motive for nursing there is contained the deep desire that no one else shall have a harder time than we do; that we shall not be cushioned away from the world like weaklings.[16]

Nurses who did not fit Dr Cabot's description but sought more professional autonomy stimulated such complaints as the following medical journal editorial that the

> recent tendency toward aggrandizement of nursing seemingly has led to the assumption of an unwarrented independence of this department from the medical organization of the hospital . . . The trained nurse is an indispensable asset, deserving of our greatest respect and appreciation: but it should be understood that, after all, she is a nurse and not a doctor. Her subordinate position in this respect should be clearly defined, and any tendency which may quite naturally develop to cross the boundary should promptly and courteously be discouraged, in her own interest as well as that of the medical profession and the patient.[17]

That same year, one Dr Bigelow, by then a proponent of education for nurses, gave a glimpse into his earlier attitude toward the nurse.

> She was a well-nigh indispensable convenience, except when she knew more than you did, when she might make you feel uncomfortable, and the male must feel psychologically superior, we are told . . . If you don't let your nurse know too

much and keep her in her place, she will remain the servile drudge of the past.[18]

Early on, nurses contributed their thoughts about the question of professionalism, identifying special knowledge and education as the key. In 1912, Annie Goodrich quoted more physicians who acknowledged nursing as a profession but advocated, as she did, better education. Goodrich recognised, even then, problems that would long remain — the fact that 'we have outgrown our system' of preparation of nurses, the need for the state to assume some definite responsibility for it, the need for universities to include nursing education and the need for higher qualifications to enter nursing schools.[19]

Hospitals were multiplying at the rate of nearly 200 per year [20] and needed staff. In order to provide it, nursing schools nearly tripled in number between 1900 and 1910.[21] Goodrich saw nursing as 'a profession struggling to protect the profession from the individual interests that would deter its members from obtaining even the minimum preparation for an efficient service to the community' and asked for some adjustment of the hospital system.[22] She recognised not only personal but social and structural requirements for professionalism.

Ten years later, Goodrich hailed the development of three national nursing organisations, a standard curriculum, and the beginnings of acceptance of nursing by Yale and other universities. Interestingly, despite her passionate advocacy of intellectual accomplishment and creativity, she recommended the passive qualities of unity, virtue and collaboration as the primary means to achieve the goal of democracy, asserting 'When we are really at one in a cause we will find that we need no leaders in the formerly accepted sense of the word . . . cooperation for creation can supersede and attain ends never possible of attainment by a society schooled for possession.'[23] Political realities proved otherwise.

Abraham Flexner had stated in his 1915 paper that 'the responsibility of the trained nurse is neither original nor final. She, too, may be described as another arm to the physician or surgeon . . . subordinates loyally her intelligence to his theory and policy.' Emily Covert disagreed. Arguing that nursing *is* a profession and does not depend on another profession, she pointed to nurses' legal liability for their actions and the growing body of knowledge taught to and by nurses. Most interesting, she used the school and rural nurses as examples of individual autonomy.[24]

In the twenties and thirties, the growth toward professionalism was primarily in the educational rather than political and societal spheres. The Standard Curriculum for Schools of Nursing, published in 1917, had been revised in 1927. Nevertheless, in 1935, Stella Goostray wrote 'The majority of our so-called schools fall far short of attaining professional educational levels and are mainly concerned with service in the hospital.'[25] In 1937, two important changes in the new Curriculum Guide provided increased flexibility and emphasized ward teaching.[26]

Still, there was evidence that focus was on the individual qualities of the nurse and that the organization and structure of practice was little questioned. 'In order to adjust well to nursing situations the nurse must possess some very definite qualities and characteristics and the effectiveness of her work is determined to a very large degree by the attitudes she has developed.' The characteristics of a nurse able to adjust well, identified by the National League for Nursing Education, included the feminine, expressive qualities of consideration, poise, co-operation, agreeability and culture.[27] This same study was the basis for Spalding's widely used 1941 textbook, *Professional Adjustments*. In it she defined nursing as an emerging profession, defined by not only the art and science of nursing but also by the spirit. The latter she described by the following traits and attributes the nurse should possess: true spiritual outlook, emotional balance, desire and capacity for hard work, courage, flexibility and others.[28] Though loyalty and obedience were no longer mentioned, creativity, leadership, initiative and advocacy had not yet emerged from the early military, self-sacrificial model.

During the same period, nursing programmes had been inching into universities, beginning at the University of Minnesota and Columbia. The *Goldmark Report* promoted professionalism through better preparation of nurses in general, and especially in public health and teaching in university settings. The subsequent Committee on Grading of Schools and its reports strengthened that impetus not only by contributing to closing weak schools but also, indirectly, by modestly improving employment of graduate nurses and practice settings.[28]

By 1928, another concern of professional self-regulation appeared in the literature. Schools had continued to multiply rapidly to approximately four times the number in 1900 and

Burgess, of the Committee on Grading, wrote 'There is serious unemployment for nurses in all parts of the country'. She proposed two answers, requiring professional initiative and attention to more than recruitment and education. One related to increasing the demand for nurses:

> It may be that the nursing profession can, through wise thought and constructive action, reorganize its methods in such a way that it can put nursing service on a self-supporting basis and utilize its immense production of new graduates in constructive and hitherto unthought-of ways.

The other strategy related to decreasing the supply of nurses:

> There has been no check on their (schools') growth. The minimum standards for nursing education are low; and the profession has as yet no effective device for doing what the medical profession has so effectively done to control the type and number of new professional recruits.[30]

Though nurses as individuals and fledgling organisations had been politically active in support of nurse licensure and practice Acts and for some health and welfare legislation since the turn of the century, the 1930s brought evidence of a gradually expanding professional ideology of involvement in political activity. By 1930 state nurses' associations had legislative committees and the American Nurses Association a small representation in Washington, DC. The ANA had supported creation of the Women's Bureau and the Sheppard-Towner Act, but by policy supported 'only measures that affect nurses and nursing, or the health and welfare of women and children'.[31] This restriction would clearly have limited confrontation with medicine, that so vehemently opposed perceived government or other inter-ference in its private practice.

As early as 1935 Goostray referred to the development of a large number of groups of health professionals, a trend that would accelerate thereafter. She expressed a speculation still heard today: 'One wonders if we had better met some of the challenging needs, there would have been the same need for so many other professional workers.'[32] She saw the major flaw and remedy in nursing education. By 1940, 161 schools had closed, but 20 per cent more nurses were graduating annually. Nevertheless, hospital days were up a like amount and, with hours of work shortening and hospital insurance growing, employment prospects for nurses looked better.[33] The needs of both armed services and civilians and the booming wartime economy and inflation placed nursing in an entirely new economic situation.

Goostray had identified in 1935 the problem of economic insecurity and widespread unemployment in nursing, and had considered the economic questions of health insurance, financing and public relations. In time, the previously rejected use of collective bargaining by a professional group was increasingly given serious discussion. As the 1940s progressed, some state nurses' associations experimented as bargaining agents.[34] But in 1948 it was estimated that not more than 3000 to 5000 of the more than 300,000 registered nurses were union members, and the great majority of nurses regarded unionisation as unacceptable.[35]

However, the ANA had had an economic security programme before the Second World War. And during the war the California State Nurses' Association had successfully acted as bargaining agent. In 1946 the ANA approved similar programmes for other states. American nurses were credited by Northrup, an industrial relations expert, with considerable initiative and foresight in the mechanics of collective bargaining and 'demonstrating how an income commensurate with professional training can be secured without sacrificing professional ethics and resorting to nonprofessional tactics'.[36]

Though economic and collective bargaining became part of nursing ideology for some, the socialisation of nurses made expression of self-concern and competition a divisive factor in the profession. From 47 per cent of eligible nurses belonging to the ANA in 1947, the number steadily dipped.[37] While circumstances of practice became of concern, they included only wages and hours, and other conditions of organised practice changed relatively little through the 1940s and 1950s. Despite efforts at collective bargaining, the nursing shortage continued to be a major problem. In 1954, the Chief of the Division of Nursing Resources, USPHS, demonstrated that graduations of nurses had kept up with population growth and nurses were working at the bedside, despite common perceptions to the contrary. She called for studies to determine the cause of the shortage, but did not implicate wages and other conditions of practice.[38]

In 1956, Witney, an economist, was not so shy about saying

that an important cause of the shortage lay in the conditions under which nurses worked, citing the number leaving nursing. 'In 1954, the average factory worker earned $323/month, or around $70 a month more than the average nurse, not to mention benefits.'[39]

In other ways nurses were changing and developing their self-images as autonomous professionals. The Second World War had been an economic boon not only to practising nurses, but also, through Federal support of the US Cadet Nurse Corps, to schools of nursing. Perhaps most important, some nurses became exposed to more autonomy, expanded roles, and, through the subsequent GI Bill, to higher education. In her influential report, *Nursing for the Future*, Esther Lucile Brown recommended: (1) that the term professional nurse be applied only to university graduates, (2) that different levels of nursing be identified, (3) that the hospital environment be changed so as to be more conducive to nurses' professional growth, and (4) nurses be paid adequate salaries to induce them to remain in nursing.[40] Her position on two levels of practice, improved salaries, and reorganisation of nursing service were similar to those of Eli Ginzberg's 1948 report *A Program for the Nursing Profession*.[41] Here was clear recognition of the importance of structure and practice as well as of selection, recruitment and individual qualities as determinants of professionalism.

In the postwar period sociologists began to study the professions. Florence Weiner suggested that nursing was emerging from an era whose ideologies have perhaps long since lost their influence. She agreed with Brown that there was an urgent need for the revision of the professional status of nurses. Reacting to the military model of nursing, she insisted that:

nursing schools, physicians, and administrators systematically recognize nurses' need for emotional security and for a clearly defined status, liberate the students' capacity to have and dispense affection as part of all nursing, which means that the effective nurse must be an emotionally mature person.[42]

Though Weiner's focus was still on improving the profession by changes in the individual, other sociologists were studying nurses' work, job tasks and boundaries, and recognising the importance of social roles. As Saunders pointed out, roles are defined in terms of collective expectations, and strain was developing as expectations of nurses, doctors and administrators became less consistent. He discussed nursing's 'Somewhat ambiguous status. The training period is long and the requirements high, but the rewards are generally low and the prestige not very great.' He also recognised some of the social and structural problems:

> It is not without significance that, even in a time of great demand for their services, the salaries of nurses remain relatively low . . . may lie in lingering notions we have about the relative capabilities of men and women . . . the rewards of the nurse, both material and psychological, are exceedingly meager.[43]

Most important, Saunders identified the issue of autonomy:

> Nursing is almost the only profession, if not the only one, in which the important decisions about what work is to be done and how it is to be done are made by people outside the profession . . . decisions under which nurses work are made by doctors.

Saunders described the isolation, bureaucratic organisation, and conservatism of nursing education and practice. In commenting on the rapidity of change in nursing, Saunders emphasised the ambivalence and conflict nurses feel between:

> ideologies about their responsibility for giving 'total patient care' . . . and being responsible for the 'total patient' . . . and the already large managerial aspect of the nursing role (that) is almost certain to increase at the expense of the more traditional elements of that role.[44]

In 1952 Pearl McIver identified the needs for change in nursing. This included increasing diversity of roles and expansion of the responsibility of the nurse as manager of nursing care provided by others less prepared. She recommended implementation through both improved nursing education and more professional responsibility and autonomy in nursing service.[45] Four years later, Saunders continued to identify problems of the profession as: role change from direct patient care to management, lack of autonomy due to external controls by doctors and hospital administrators and changes in images and expectations of the profession, both by nurses and others. He identified growing recognition of nurses as technically competent professionals who 'Increasingly expect to work in a relationship of colleague equality'.[46]

Bennis and Benne also identified role conflict and confusion in their study of the professional nurse in the outpatient department. They suggested:

> taking a close look at the idealized image to see if it is realistically relevant to our working situation . . . in our experience, nurses suffer too much guilt and anguish from having to live up to internalized canons that are outdated, and nostalgic principles which do not have high relevance to their modern work situation.[47]

In the 1960s and 1970s the familiar problems of role conflict and professional dominance continued to be addressed in the literature. Aydelotte and Hudson wrote of the conflict engendered by physician dominance of the total nurse-patient-doctor situation, the problem of the severe nurse shortage, doubts about nurses' ability to function more autonomously and about the system's ability to treat them more equitably. But they did plead for detailed analysis of the setting and structure of practice.[48] Ashley later wryly observed, 'Dominant influences in health care will not yield to the private and quiet pleas of pacifying women: powerful, male dominated groups, economically motivated, will not be reasonable with their interests and status threatened.'[49]

In 1945 the AMA House of Delegates, in discussing nursing education, had declared its authority:

> The problem is so definitely one of multiple jurisdictional interest and responsibility in which the medical profession as well as hospital management have a major part and obligation to the public to use the weight of their experience and authority in assisting to bring about the most perfect program possible in the nursing field.[50]

By 1962, the AMA, though obviously asserting its continuing concern with nursing, recognised nursing's 'separate and distinct professional status' and offered support and understanding of all levels of nursing, while avoiding the brewing entry-level controversy.[51]

Several major new influences on nursing professionalisation developed in the 1960s and 1970s, particularly the civil rights, anti-war, anti-poverty, women's movements and massive Federal involvement in health care and education. The latter two combined to directly affect nursing. Growing numbers of women, especially wives and mothers who hadn't previously sought careers, found both encouragement and financial assistance to enter nursing. The expanding community colleges made low cost education available, and additional public support of health care for the elderly and underserved increased the demand for nurses.

The Nurse Training Act of 1964 and its extensions in the Health Manpower Act of 1968, and thereafter in the early 1970s, authorised previously unheard of amounts of financial assistance for nursing schools and students. This contributed to strengthening of diploma and associate degree programmes and maintenance of the *status quo* in nursing education at a time when the ANA, in 1965, first endorsed the baccalaureate degree for entry into practice. The relative lack of power of the ANA in the area of policy making was also demonstrated in 1964, with rejection of its recommendation that 'Special emphasis must be given to the basic baccalaureate degree programs.'[52] Again, in 1968, nursing leaders were disappointed. Rozella Schlotfeldt, Chair of the ANA Commission on Education, ANA, wrote Senator Lister Hill, Chair of Committee on Labour and Public Welfare, expressing enthusiasm for the proposed extension of basic support grants to baccalaureate programmes, but 'We are very concerned that Section 231 of Title II would permit the Commissioner of Education to name a state agency as the accrediting body for the purpose of determining eligibility for federal funding.'[53] The law did not require national accreditation of schools.

The provisions of the Medicare and Medicaid legislation, provided federally supported health care for the elderly and poor, passed the preceding year, also strengthened the position of hospitals and medicine by increasing demands for their services and providing cost-plus reimbursement. Though nursing wages also rose with the time, there was little impetus to increase professional autonomy until escalating costs forced new scrutiny of the health care system.

In an effort to improve access to and restrain costs of health care, Federal legislation of the 1970s encouraged educational programmes to prepare nurses for expanded roles, such as nurse practitioner, and practice settings, such as HMOs and community care. This and the rise of consumerism produced demands for more involvement by clients in their own health care, such as home births, and enthusiasm among some nurses for more independent practice and for assuming the role of patient advocate. In a bicentennial address, Gabrielson, President of the ANA, identified nursing as the conscience of the health care system and a leader in securing rights of human beings.

Federal efforts to eliminate the still perceived nursing shortage included, in addition to assistance to all levels of nurse training programmes, traineeships for preparation of nurse faculty and administrators, school building construction, leadership development through research grants and the nurse scientist programme.[54] Professional autonomy was undoubtedly advanced by this expansion of educated, university-based leadership and also by the requirements in practice for more specialisation and technical competence and for more personalised patient care. However, achievement of the political goals of creating a large supply of relatively inexpensive nurses fostered expanding associate degree and continuing diploma education which was problematic for those nursing leaders promoting professional autonomy.

Freidson said of nursing:

> Like many others, the occupation is composed of a small proportion of policy makers, supervisors, and teaching nurses dedicated to professionalization striving to mobilize a heterogeneous and shifting corps of often casual and transient skilled workers . . .[55]

He saw nursing's struggle toward professionalism as related to 'motivation to see oneself as an active, creative worker of some importance who can adopt a therapeutic rather than a custodial attitude toward the patient'.[56] He said 'the nurse is not fully professional . . . it's a would-be profession, and if only because of the strength of the medical profession, is unlikely to attain full professional status'.[57]

Etzioni also saw nursing as less than a full profession, based on lack of a body of knowledge relevant to patient care and developed by nurses.In addition, he, like Freidson, saw social and structural problems; 'nurses' caste-like separation from physicians must give way to the colleagueship that now prevails among the various medical specialities'.[58] He suggested that, rather than as manager or as physician-surrogate, a return to the bedside might offer the best prospects of professional autonomy 'if she could persuade the physician that her skills are of professional caliber comparable to his own'.[59] Advocates of primary nursing and certified advanced practice share this thinking.

In 1982, Richard Hall, a sociologist specialising in theory of professions and organisations, described analyses of professions as being approached in two ways. The traditional, attribute approach focused on characteristics of occupations and individuals. Hall felt the other approach, developed by Freidson and Johnson and based on acquisition and use of power in the larger social structure, is clearly dominant. This approach emphasises:

> the ability to obtain and maintain professional status (that) is closely related to concrete occupational strategies, as well as wider social forces and arrangements of power. That is, there is both an internal and external dynamic of professionalism.[60]

Hall went on to comment that the professional model seems to be very much on the minds of people in fields striving to become truly professional, fields such as nursing. Hall concluded that:

> among sociologists concerned with the nature of professions, there is near concensus that power is the critical defining characteristic. Power provides a profession with the capacity to have legislation passed which protects its areas of practice. Power provides the capacity to establish agreed upon credentials. Power provides the capacity to demand and receive reasonable levels of compensation.[61]

Hall also identified the strains of employed professional work, especially for nurses who work directly with other professional groups who are themselves concerned with issues of domain of practice, credentials, standards and compensation. He, again, saw power as the key in dealing with employing organisations and other professions.

With the 1970s and 1980s came not only increasing attention to the environmental or structural aspects of professionalisation, but also re-examination of the more obvious and traditional individual values and attitudes. Winslow examined the developing changes in nursing ethics, identifying the two basic metaphors for nursing most often espoused by leaders and having most obvious effects on education and practice. The first is the military metaphor, of nursing in the battle against disease and associated with virtues such as loyalty and norms of obedience to and maintainance of confidence in authority figures. The second metaphor is nursing as advocacy of patients' rights, an essentially legal metaphor and associated with virtues such as courage and norms such as defence of the patient against infringement of rights.

Winslow sagely commented 'It would be surprising if professional nursing had not early adapted the metaphor of military service,'[62] based as it is on Florence Nightingale's experiences in the Crimean War and Victorian concepts of acceptable behaviour for women. Both fostered conformity, deference to rank, obedience and the key virtue, loyalty . . . not autonomy. Though loyalty of the nurse meant faithful and self-sacrificial care of patients, 'most of the discussions of loyalty were occupied more with another concern; the protection of confidence in the health care effort'.[63]

Joyce Thompson has also expressed concern for both ethical problems and the social context within which nurses practise and make decisions in health and illness care particularly as employees in bureaucratic institutions. She asserted 'To be professional is to be ethical; to be ethical is to be autonomous. Nurses need to maintain or gain (or regain) control over their own practice and their profession.'[64]

The issue of the boundary between nursing and other groups, especially medicine, is increasingly discussed. McClosky argues that, though nurse practitioners can undertake without difficulty about two-thirds the range of work normally allotted to a general practitioner doctor, professional enhancement of nurses in the US will flow from differentiation from physicians, hospitals and the traditional female role.[65] Hicks, considering the same subject in Australia, pointed out 'Chiropractic achieved political legitimation not by accepting the doctor's science but by matching their public acceptability.'[66]

In the mid 1980s there is ample evidence that at least nursing leadership recognises the imperative to address issues such as autonomy, power and the structural as well as individual attributes necessary to achieve nursing professionalism. Hunter and Berger wrote:

> While historic strategies such as defining a knowledge base, generating nursing research, building a professional association, and bargaining collectively have moved nurses toward professional self-determination, they have been proven necessary but insufficient conditions of autonomy. The missing component has been a strategic understanding of the role of public policy in advancing professional ideals . . .
> Nurses' ability in the future to deal with critical policy questions and manifest their political potential may well lie in how effectively nursing leaders learn to translate policy issues into symbols relating to the fundamental concerns of working nurses.[67]

A recent survey of nursing administrators and deans reflected recognition by these leaders of the growing importance of and need for nursing influence on health policy.[68,69] The political strategies identified as most successful were communicating and collaborating with not only legislators but also peers and consumer coalitions. Milio subsequently reaffirmed nursing's growing concerns about effects of the rapidly changing controls, structure and funding of the health care system. She, also, recommended organisation, analysis, communication and collaboration with public and allies. She acknowledged the relatively 'poor and powerless' position of nursing but the potential for leaders to influence health policy making.[70]

Judith Ryan, Executive Director of ANA, has also expressed the need for nurses to be given experience in the policy arena and articulated the goal for the organisation to define ways in which nurses will have to organise in order to deliver their services, to establish standards for services and guidelines for preparation of nurses and to decide how services will be financed.[71]

Other strategies and proposals for addressing these issues are being developed. Stiller described an example of learning from experience:

> in the early sixties reimbursable home care was decided by compromising forces between the AMA, AHA and interest

groups in favor of universal care for the elderly . . . Now, twenty years later, we are still struggling with the fact that what is deemed reimbursable is not necessarily public health nursing.[72]

Regulations and policy are shaping practice rather than nursing shaping policy.

A nurse who is a Maryland legislator, Marilyn Goldwater, has succeeded in shaping policy and legislation, instituting a comprehensive study of nursing issues, direct reimbursement for nurses and actively influencing the 10 per cent of Bills in the Maryland Legislature that are health related.[73] Experience has taught Goldwater that:

A serious roadblock to use of power is reluctance of individuals within the profession to assert themselves or to align themselves with organizations that can exert the power needed to effect change . . . When a governmental body becomes convinced that a group speaks with the force of knowledge and authority, that group has gained either a powerful ally or a nervous antagonist. Either way, the concerns of the organization will become the concerns of the government.[74]

The strength and activity of organised nursing is also necessary to increase autonomy and nursing professionalisation. Establishment of a Washington office in 1951 and increasing activity of the Committee on Economic and General Welfare reflected efforts of the ANA to increase nursing's power. Activities included support for equal pay for equal work, minority rights and improvement of pay and working conditions.[75] State nurses' associations began organising political action committees in 1974, and N-CAP was organised by the ANA in 1976. Though these are separate from their parent organisations, they do co-operate.[76] Hall maintained that 'The professional association would appear to be the only real source of the power for establishing nursing as a profession and supporting its members . . .'[77]

Smith, in considering the professional goals of autonomy and authority, raises an important question about the role of nursing organisations. She pointed out that the ANA has been sharpening its image as a labour organisation in the past decade, but that activity conflicts with other efforts to be a multipurpose

170

professional organisation. Whether ANA can be both is a major issue, she says, and 'the question of who will address national issues when states choose to go their own ways has not yet been resolved'.[78]

Smith went on to support the need for structural changes in the relationship of nursing to major social institutions. 'The lesson of the last quarter century is that nursing has not become more autonomous or influential in terms of health policy decisions. Nursing's public image remains that of physician's helpmate.' She predicted that collective bargaining is unlikely to make nurses more autonomous or in control of health policy, and that 'Recognition as a profession rather than an occupation may rest on other bases — for example, specialization, entrepreneurship, and public expressions of nursing symbols, values and dogma.'[79]

Better preparation of nursing administrators is suggested as another avenue toward recognition of nursing as a profession. Fralic endorsed a concept of nursing professionalism that includes recognition of not only individual ideology and skills, but also relationships with other professions and the system in order to produce leaders for nursing from the nursing profession — not to have them developed and superimposed from outside nursing (business, management, administration, etc.). 'The growth and support of nursing as a practice discipline will depend on how well we develop our own nurse administrators.'[80]

Each of the five themes emerging from the hearings of the National Commission on Nursing in 1981 requires understanding of nursing as more than a noble calling practised by dedicated individuals. Each theme emphasises nursing as a more autonomous part of a complex system of social relationships. The themes included: status and image of nursing, interface of nursing education and practice, effective nursing management of the nursing resource, relationships among nursing, medical staff and health care administrators and maturation of nursing as a self-determining profession.[81]

This paper has presented an overview of the historical development of the ideology of nursing professionalism. Nursing literature since 1902 has reflected the gradual and accelerating shift away from the traditional, attribute approach, viewing professionalism in terms of individual attributes and characteristics that, once internalised through education, will be demonstrated regardless of subsequent circumstances of practice. Writings and activities of nursing leaders, particularly

171

in the past 25 years, have increasingly adopted the power perspective of professionalism. Viewing the emerging nursing profession in relation to other occupational groups and the larger social structure has brought into focus concerns with autonomy, power and political activity.

NOTES

1. Eliot Freidson, *Professional dominance: the social structure of medical care* (Atherton Press, New York, 1970), p.49.

2. Ibid., p.60.

3. Lucie Young Kelly, *Dimensions of professional nursing*, 5th edn (Macmillan, New York, 1985).

4. G. Bixler and R. Bixler, 'The professional status of nursing', *American Journal of Nursing* (AJN), 45 (9) (1945), pp.730–5.

5. Abraham Flexner, 'Is social work a profession?', *School and Society*, 1, 26 (1915), pp.901–11.

6. F. Lewis and M. Batey, 'Clarifying autonomy and accountability in nursing service', *Journal of Nursing Administration*, 12 (10) (1982), pp.10–15.

7. R. Morantz and S. Zschoche, 'Professionalism, feminism and gender roles' in J. Leavitt (ed.), *Women and health in America* (University of Wisconsin Press, Madison, Wi., 1984), p.407.

8. Freidson, *Professional dominance*, pp.63–4.

9. Linda Richards,'The entrance of the nursing profession into reform and protective work', *AJN*, 2 (May 1902), pp.59–3.

10. Lavinia Dock, *A history of nursing* (Putnams, New York, 1912).

11. Laurie Glass, 'Safeguarding society's welfare: nursing's political history', *Nursing Success Today*, 1 (4) (1984), pp.39–40.

12. Dock, *A history of nursing*, pp.972–3.

13. Ibid., pp.973–5.

14. A. Worcester, 'Is nursing really a profession?', *AJN*, 2 (August 1902), pp.908–17.

15. J. Ashley, *Hospitals, paternalism and the role of the nurses* (Teachers College Press, New York, 1976), p.100.

16. Richard Cabot, 'The motive of nursing', *Boston Medical Surgical Journal*, 190 (9) (1923), pp.355–7.

17. Leonard Freeman, 'Nurse vs. doctor', *Surgery, Gynecology and Obstetrics*, 45 (November 1927), pp.711–12.

18. George Bigelow, 'The profession of nursing', *Boston Medical Surgical Journal*, 196 (9) (1927), pp.355–7.

19. Annie Goodrich, 'The complete nurse', *AJN*, 12 (1912), pp.777–82.

20. Stella Goostray, 'What lies ahead for the nursing profession?' *AJN*, 35 (8) (1935), pp.765–71.

21. May Burgess, 'Where does nursing want to go?', *AJN*, 28 (5) (1928), pp.481–5.

22. Goodrich, 'The complete nurse', p.780.

23. Annie Goodrich, 'The objective of the nurse in a democracy', *AJN*, 22 (9) (1922), pp.1005-11.

24. Emily Covert, 'Is nursing a profession?', *AJN*, 18 (November 1917), pp.107–8.

25. Goostray, 'What lies ahead for the nursing profession?', p.766.

26. Norma Anderson, 'The historical development of American nursing education', *Journal of Nursing Education*, 20 (1) (1981), pp.18–35.

27. Laura Eads, 'Characteristics of a nurse able to adjust well to nursing situations', *AJN*, 36 (7) (1936), pp.705–15.

28. E. Spalding, *Professional adjustments in nursing* (Lippincott, New York, 1941), p.99.

29. Anderson, 'The historical development of American nursing education', p.28.

30. Burgess, 'Where does nursing want to go?, pp.484–5.

31. Clara Noyes, 'Federal legislation and the American Nurses' Association', *AJN*, 30 (4) (1930), pp.425–9.

32. Goostray, 'What lies ahead for the nursing profession?', p.767.

33. 'Professional drifts and shifts', *AJN*, 41 (1) (1941), pp.2–8.

34. William Scott, 'Shall professional nurses become collective bargaining agents for their members?', *AJN*, 44 (3) (1944), pp.231–2.

35. Herbert Northrup, 'Collective bargaining and the professions', *AJN*, 48 (3) (1948), pp.141–2.

36. Ibid., p.144.

37. 'Some international trends', *AJN*, 47 (5) (1947), p.359.

38. Margaret Arnstein, 'Setting the record straight: 1954', *Nursing Outlook*, vol.2 (June 1984).

39. Fred Witney, 'Is nursing meeting its obligation to society?', *AJN*, 56 (9) (1956), pp.1127–31.

40. Esther L. Brown, *Nursing for the future: a report prepared for the National Nursing Council* (Russell Sage Foundation, New York, 1948).

41. Anderson, 'The historical development of nursing education', p.30.

42. Florence Weiner, 'Professional consequences of the nurse's occupational status', *AJN*, 51 (10) (1951), pp.614–17.

43. Lyle Saunders, 'The changing role of nurses', *AJN*, 54 (9) (1954), pp.1094–5.

44. Ibid., p.1097.

45. Pearl McIver, 'Nursing moves forward', *AJN*, 52 (7) (1952), pp.821–3.

46. Lyle Saunders, 'Permanence and change', *AJN*, 58 (7) (1958), p.972.

47. Kenneth Benne and Warren Bennis, 'Role confusion and role conflict in nursing: the role of the professional nurse', *AJN*, 59 (2) (1959), pp.196–8.

48. M. Aydelotte and W. Hudson, 'A socio-engineering problem — the nursing profession', *Nursing Outlook*, 10 (1) (1962), pp.20–23.

49. Ashley, *Hospitals, paternalism and the role of the nurses*, p.133.

50. Ibid.,p.122.

51. 'Objectives and program of the AMA Committee on Nursing',

Journal of the American Medical Association, 181 (4 August 1962), p.430.

52. Surgeon General's Consultant Group on Nursing. Archives of the American Nurses' Association, Folder 33 (1963), American Nurses' Association, Kansas City, Missouri (AMA Archives)

53. R. Schlotfeldt to L. Hill (4 April 1968), AMA archives.

54. Health Manpower Act of 1968, United States Public Law #90–490.

55. Freidson, *Professional dominance*, p.21.

56. Ibid., p.27.

57. Ibid., p.21.

58. A. Etzioni, *The semi-professionals and their organization* (Free Press, New York, 1969), p.76.

59. Ibid., p.71.

60. Richard Hall, 'The professions employed professionals, and the professional association' in *Professionalism and the empowerment of nursing: papers presented at the 53rd Convention of the American Nurses' Association* (The Association, Washington, DC, 1982).

61. Ibid., p.13.

62. Gerald R. Winslow, 'From loyalty to advocacy: a new metaphor for nursing', *The Hastings Center Report* (June 1984), p.32.

63. Ibid., p.33.

64. Joyce Thompson, 'Professionalism and the empowerment of nursing: conflicting loyalties of nurses working in bureaucratic settings', *American Nurses' Association Publication* #G–157–27–37 (1982).

65. J. C. McClosky, 'The professionalization of nursing, United States and England', *International Nursing Review*, 28 (2) (1981), pp.40–47.

66. Neville Hicks, 'The history and politics of legislation for nursing status', *Australian Journal of Advanced Nursing*, 2 (3) (1985), pp.47–55.

67. Patricia Hunter and Karen Berger, 'Nurses and the political arena: lobbying for professional impact', *Nursing Administration Quarterly*, 8 (4) (1984), pp.66–79.

68. S. Archer and P. Goehner, 'Acquiring political clout: guidelines for nurse administrators', *The Journal of Nursing Administration*, 11 (11–12) (1981), pp.49–55.

69. S. Archer, 'Study of nurse administrators' political participation', *Western Journal of Nursing Research*, 1 (1983), pp.65–75.

70. Nancy Milio, 'The realities of policy making: can nurses have an impact?', *The Journal of Nursing Administration*, 14 (3) (1984), pp.18–23.

71. Judith Ryan, 'Judith Ryan shares thoughts with Missouri nurses', *The Missouri Nurse*, 54 (2) (1985), pp.8–10.

72. Susan Stiller, 'Shaping the future of nurses through political awareness and action', *Connecticut Nursing News*, 58 (5) (1985), p.3.

73. Marilyn Goldwater, 'Influencing health policy through the political process', *Florida Nurse*, 31 (9) (1985), pp.11–23.

74. Marilyn Goldwater, 'Political power for nurse practitioners', *Nurse Practitioner*, 9 (11) (1984), pp.44–9.

75. *The nature and scope of ANA economic and general welfare policy*

(American Nurses' Association, Kansas City, Missouri, 1985).

76. Gerry Cadenhead, 'PACs — what they are and what they do', *Missouri RN*, 45 (2) (1983), pp.16–17.

77. Hall, 'The professions employed professionals, and the professional associations', p.13.

78. Gloria Smith, 'Nursing power: the political experience', *The Oklahoma Nurse* (19–21 December 1985), p.19.

79. Ibid., pp.19–20.

80. Maryann Fralic, 'Preferred patterns of preparation: the nurse executive role', unpublished paper presented at the National League for Nursing, Second Nurse Educator Conference (1986).

81. Ruth B. Fine, 'The supply and demand of nursing administrators', *Nursing and Health Care* (January 1983), p.10.

11

Profit and Loss and the Hospital Nurse

Christopher Maggs

INTRODUCTION

Too often, the history of nursing has failed to take account of wider social events and contexts, and the development of modern nursing is frequently portrayed in isolation from the mainstream of society. For example, some nurse historians appear to have overlooked, in their concern with professionalisation, the obvious fact that nursing is an economic activity. Not only is it paid work but numbers of nurses work and train in hospitals and other institutions, which were built at considerable expense and which continue to interact with the local economies in significant ways. An analysis of this relationship between hospital nursing and the economy may enhance our understanding of the way in which modern nursing developed. This chapter looks at one provincial English hospital in the period 1850–80 in order to examine that relationship and extend our understanding of the development of nursing in the nineteenth century.

That health (or conversely, ill-health) is an industry or sector of the economy is almost a truism. As Hamilton, writing of the growth of non-profit making voluntary sector health care in the United States in the 1960s, argued, 'the local hospital is the town's biggest employer and operates the largest hotel, laundry, pharmacy and restaurant; collectively, hospitals make up one of the country's largest industries and are a vital cog in the nation's economic structure'.[1] That was also the case for England and Wales in the interwar and immediate postwar years.[2] Abel-Smith, in his study of the development of hospitals in England and Wales, also draws attention to the relationship between economic activity and the growth and viability of hospitals in the nineteenth and early twentieth centuries.[3]

It is also the case that the hospital is an ideological metaphor, in which systems of control are constructed which operate not simply to cure or to treat but to manage, to classify and to maintain.[4] Once established — and that was not always a straightforward task[5] — the overriding function of the hospital was to ensure its own survival; those who worked in it were adjuncts of that function. Thus, the constant concern of lay administrators was economic viability; all other characteristics which made up the hospital were but elements in an equation of profit and loss. Into that arena came the 'new nurses', at first an unwelcome additional burden on the financial well being of the hospital, and eventually an agent of its survival. In order that that might be achieved, structures were evolved or borrowed from other institutions, such as the business firm and the factory; the asylum; and the prison. For example, time discipline; book-keeping and stock control; and a division of labour superficially based on skill but having more to do with class and gender power relations. The hospital so closely identified with business and commerce that a group of doctors — consultant, registrars, junior and students — became known as a 'firm'.

THE GROWTH OF THE VOLUNTARY HOSPITALS

The first modern phase of growth of hospitals took place in England in the eighteenth century. The 'famous names' of the hospital world were founded in this period. For example, the Westminster; Guy's; St George's; the London and the Middlesex were all opened between 1720 and 1745. Outside London, 28 hospitals were commissioned between 1730 and 1800, beginning with Winchester (1736); Bath General (1742); Royal Devon and Exeter (1743); Manchester Royal Infirmary (1752) and Sheffield Royal Infirmary (1797). Many were founded by individuals, as in the case of Thomas Guy and Guy's Hospital, London, or by local groups of concerned citizens, as in the case of the Royal Devon and Exeter which Ruth Hawker outlines in her contribution in this volume.[6]

In general, this early phase in hospital growth was the direct result of the increased prosperity of the middle classes, a wealth based on mercantile capitalism. In a period of relative prosperity, there was a perception of a widening gap opening up between the rich — many newly rich — and the poor. That prompted a resurgence of Christian humanitarianism which was expressed in increased charitable endeavours, of which founding hospitals was but one example.[7] There is little doubt of the wealth of many of the founders of these early hospitals. Thomas Guy may be an exceptional case but his story none the less offers insights into this period. He had been a Lombard Street bookseller who, unlike many, made a fortune 'by the sale of Bibles, Seamen's tickets and South Sea Bubble Stock'.[8] He turned his fortune, which amounted to nearly a quarter of a million eighteenth-century pounds, into an endowment for the hospital which has since borne his name.

Unlike the hospices and earlier hospitals, these 'new' hospitals were not for paupers but for the industrious poor and, in particular, for the urban poor. The London (1740) was set up to help 'in particular, the manufacturers and merchant seamen together with their families'.[9] The links between commerce and hospital growth are shown in many of the provincial hospitals. For example, the Bristol General Hospital (1737) was set up to provide hospital facilities for those engaged in the slave triangle trade using part of the personal fortune of one man actively involved in it, John Elbridge, a quaker and collector of customs.[10] Liverpool's first hospital was opened in 1749 and closely associated with the trade in that port. This development, providing health care in hospitals to those engaged in wealth creation in order to return them as quickly as possible to the labour force, was to be enshrined and exaggerated in the welfare and medical provisions which resulted from the Poor Law Amendment Act of 1834.

However, the total number of inpatients treated in these new hospitals was relatively small. Census data, notoriously unreliable, suggest that in 1800 there were less than 3,000 inpatients in England and Wales; at the census date in 1851, that total had risen to approximately 7,600.[11] Of course, such data cannot tell us about the total number of patients who passed through the hospitals; in the absence of data concerning turnover, length of stay and bed occupancy, we are left very much in the dark about this period.

By 1861, however, the position had very much altered. Whilst inpatient data from this period are still vague and difficult to interpret,[12] an impression of the rate of the expansion in hospital provision comes from data on available hospital beds. In 1861, there were approximately 65,000 hospital beds for the physically ill in England and Wales — of which about 15,000 were in the voluntary hospitals. By 1891, the voluntary sector provided 29,520 beds and this rose to 56,550 in 1921. This expansion in beds, whilst still a relatively small part of the total hospital provision in England and Wales, was remarkable as was the growth of its relative share of the total provision. In 1861 there were 23 teaching hospitals; 25 in 1938. But there were 130 voluntary hospitals in 1861; 385 in 1891; 530 in 1911 and by 1921 the total was 616.[13]

That second phase of hospital expansion began in the mid-nineteenth century, coinciding with and produced by the return to relative economic stability, now based on a new system — industrial capitalism. This expansion came about by a combination of a number of factors. Demographic change, in particular in the urban areas, influenced the provision of hospitals, although there was no correlation between population growth and national and regional bed provision. London had more beds for the physically ill per 1,000 heads of population than any other area throughout the nineteenth and much of the twentieth centuries. The changes in medical science and medical fashion accounted for some of the expansion, in particular in the rise of the specialist institutions such as St Mark's Hospital, London, which treated colono-rectal diseases. In the more rural areas, small hospitals were opened by local 'general practitioners' in an attempt to safeguard their incomes from competition from the larger voluntary hospitals in nearby towns and cities which had 'consultants' on their staffs.[14]

HOSPITAL ADMINISTRATION AND FINANCING

In general, voluntary hospitals fell into one of two types so far as finances. The first group were the endowed hospitals, such as Guy's, which had large legacies and which, if managed wisely, could provide income both for maintenance and for upgrading and possibly for expansion. Most voluntary hospitals were, however, not endowed but depended on subscriptions and donations. The Royal South Hants Infirmary in Southampton, England, was one provincial voluntary hospital heavily dependent on income from subscribers.

179

Founded in 1838 as a 'casualty Ward' following a devastating fire in the town, the Royal South Hants Infirmary (RSH) expanded in 1844 when the institution moved into a purpose-built infirmary which could 'accommodate 45 Patients, 1,000 cubic feet of air being provided for each Patient'.[15] It was from the first always in financial straits. Income derived from three major sources. First, there was the system of subscriptions; members of the local community, mainly the wealthy and the middle class, annually paid the sum of one guinea (later, two) and became Governors of the hospital. Payment of a single sum of £21 (nineteenth-century pounds) or more entitled the person to become a governor for life. In return, subscribers were given the right to recommend one inpatient or three outpatients per year for each guinea subscribed. (The Management Committee had decided, following an extensive review in 1859, not to institute the 'ticket system' which other hospitals were said to use.) The second source of income came from donations, straightforward gifts to the hospital. Finally, the hospital also held investments, either purchased by the Management Committee or left to the hospital in the will of a local dignitary or philanthropist.

One source of income which never managed to become a major contribution was that derived from patients themselves. The total income derived from patients never amounted to more than 5 per cent of the total income in any one year throughout the period and, indeed, that proportion declined steadily over the century.

In the main, those payments were made not by the patients themselves but by their employers. The rules of the RSH prohibited the admission of certain employees including domestic servants:

Until the Institution shall be in possession of considerable annual income, no apprentice or domestic servant (except servants of Annual Subscribers of not less than Three Guineas) shall be admitted, unless the recommending Governor shall engage to pay one shilling daily for his, or her, subsistence in the Infirmary.[16]

The same rules also made it clear which categories of patients would be liable to contribute towards their care: 'members of clubs, pensioners, inhabitants of alms-houses receiving salaries, and others in similar circumstances, shall be required to make some weekly payment whilst resident in the Infirmary'.[17]

In 1855, the total income of the RSH amounted to £2,473. Thirty-six per cent (£883 8s 6d) came from subscriptions; 25 per cent (£613 14s 11d) from donations and approximately 30 per cent (£742) from investment income. The remainder was made up of legacies, payments by patients and employers and by the sale of slops from the hospital kitchen. By 1862, income had risen to £3,010 17s 10d of which 38 per cent derived from subscriptions and 22 per cent from donations.

The investment patterns of the mid-nineteenth century are reflected in the investments made on behalf of the RSH. Portfolios included railways, consols and dock schemes. Investment in government stock continued throughout the period; it did have a measure of long-term attractiveness but given its relatively poor rate of return, this investment was probably the result of codicils within specific bequests rather than investment choice.

Much of this investment was in local stock, including South Western Railway which had its terminus in Southampton Docks or the Southampton Dock Company itself. In 1856, £1,200 of South Western Railway debentures provided a dividend of £50; in the same year, £1,253 12s 3d worth of consols brought in £35 5s 3d. Over the next six years the Management Committee of the RSH sold its holdings in the railway, with the last of the Bills being sold in 1862 for £306 6s. That same year, the dividends from waterworks and docks holdings amounted to only £8 and £10 respectively. The share boom had come to a temporary halt and the flush of wealth created by the railway mania was fading from the face of the economy.

However, even if the amount raised by investments was relatively small when compared with that derived from subscriptions and donations, the two areas were closely connected as can be seen from the interest shown in the hospital by the P & O Company, which operated both passenger and cargo services from Southampton Docks. As in other ports such as Bristol, Liverpool and London, there was a need for hospital and accident facilities for both passengers and crew members. The company was a 'Life Governor' of the RSH, and paid £21 each year through its agent, Captain Engledue who was also appointed Vice-President of the Infirmary. Donations were also received from the company and collections were taken regularly on board the ships by Captain Engledue and his fellow captains. In 1861, the amount raised by collections on P & O ships came to more than £112. If we consider that the entire cost of wages for nurses, porters and domestic servants (excluding the matron who was paid £48 15s and the house surgeon who received £50) came to £179 9s 5d that year, we can measure the importance of such donations to the institution. The association between Captain Engledue, on behalf of the company, and the hospital brought benefits in turn to P & O; in 1859, a total of 91 seamen were treated as inpatients by the hospital.

The mutuality of interest which this case demonstrates was not unusual nor in any way improper; what it does illustrate are some of the very close links which existed between the hospital and the local economy. Those links were, of course, extended by the personal involvement, as subscribers, Life Governors and members of the Management Committee, by local businessmen and families who employed numbers of servants and other workers.

The interaction between the hospital as a business and the local economy may also be shown in the first year of the hospital's existence. Then a local chemist, perhaps with an eye to future contracts, offered to supply gratis all medicines to the infirmary in its first year of operations. The offer was accepted, but we do not know whether that chemist received subsequent contracts.[18] Many other local firms, including manufacturing and commercial enterprises as well as solicitors and retailers were individual or company subscribers. Some firms, for example Dixon and Cardus, put up collection boxes on their premises so that their workmen might contribute to the hospital. They also encouraged their workmen to pay in regular weekly subscriptions to the treasurer.

It will have become apparent that the financial position of the hospital, and many like it,[19] which relied on uncertain public support for the bulk of its income must always have been precarious. As the Management Committee of the RSH recorded in its *Annual Report for 1860*, 'in common with all other hospitals, a very large portion of the income of the Infirmary is derived from uncertain sources'.[20] In a year when total income amounted to approximately £3,668, almost a third had to be made up from exceedingly precarious sources — legacies, small gifts of money, proceeds from concerts and similar fund raising efforts. As an example of the lengths to which the Management

Committee was forced to go to get donations, a visit to South-ampton Docks in 1860 by the Great Eastern Steamship was used as an opportunity to have a collection among sightseers. The event raised nearly £75, very welcome in view of the fact that that was the amount spent on wines and spirits — crucial to the medical care then available in the hospital.[21] And it was not just money which helped to keep the hospital afloat. Gifts of equip-ment, from water beds and pillows to easy chairs for the dayrooms, were vital to the viability of the institution.

Fund-raising by bazaars, church appeals and concerts, etc., also served to introduce new or potential subscribers, important because of the relatively high 'drop out' rate amongst subscribers in this period. However, as all fund-raisers will know, income from such events is sensitive to fluctuations in both the local and the national economy. In times of high unemployment, a drop in living standards, or price inflation, income from fund raising often fell. Later in the century such indiscriminate charity giving also came in for attack by the Charity Organisation Society. In calling for a House of Lords committee of investigation into the income and expenditure of the London voluntary hospitals (and by implication, all voluntary hospitals), the COS pointed out that the annual deficit of the London voluntary hospitals had risen from £32,000 in 1877 to £100,000 in 1899, with at least 2,000 beds closed as a direct result.[22]

In that context, the character of the person responsible for the financial management of the hospital was central. But so was that of the person who 'collected' the subscriptions and donations, the man who actually handled much of the money which the hospital received. The work of the treasurer was part accountant and part publicist. A good treasurer could help raise income by advertising 'cure rates' or bed occupancy figures in the local press and in his reports. The fraudulent collector, on the other hand, could wipe out most of a year's income by running off with the collections, as sometimes happened. In an attempt to safeguard itself against that possibility, the RSH, in keeping with other hospitals, gave the post of collector either to someone who purchased it — and hence had a stake in maintaining his reputation — or to the nominee of one of the influential subscribers or member of the Management Committee, thus insuring against fraud. That both the treasurer and collector posts could be in the gift of a few powerful people was a cause of concern to some management committees. As a consequence of this nepotism and to prevent abuses resulting from it in the day-to-day running of the institution, many local hospitals set up visiting committees, along the lines of those organised for the prisons and the workhouses.

Rarely did the treasurer involve himself in medical or clinical matters, at least directly. Provided the house surgeon followed the rules of the hospital and provided no additional expense was incurred, day-to-day medical decisions were made by the doctors.[23] Occasionally, the treasurer did intervene. In 1858, for example, the number of potential inpatients increased beyond the bed-occupancy capability of the hospital. In other words, too many patients were chasing too few beds. On the advice of the treasurer, the Committee stepped in and restricted admissions to the hospital. It did this despite the house surgeon's wish to enter all he saw fit to admit, and despite the fact that many of those seeking admission came with a recommendation from important subscribers. A waiting list was thus created, incidentally creating increased demand for beds which in turn helped to generate increased income, and which all added to the developing status and power of the professional lay administrator.

However, despite an increasing professionalism among administrators, they remained imbued with old values, in particular the need to balance the books and if possible create a surplus against future need. Hard-pressed hospital secretaries, as they generally became known, resorted to what might be called 'creative accounting' in their often desperate attempts to increase income or disguise expenditure. As Robert Pinker has noted, many administrators 'presented their statistics more with the aim of raising additional funds than accounting for those they had already received and spent'.[24] One particular accounting method used by such administrators was the 'mystery' of the 'Capital and Current Accounts'.[25] For example, a new boiler could be included under 'Extraordinary Expenditure' and thus reduce the average cost per bed that year, which was based on 'Ordinary Expenditure'.[26] Cost per bed and bed-occupancy rates were crucial statistics for presentation to the public and subscribers to convince them that the hospital was running efficiently. On the other hand, certain donations could be described in the administrator's report as 'special' and subsequently omitted from the heading 'Income on Maintenance Account'. This somewhat esoteric-sounding practice could, at a stroke, reduce on paper the total current income and thus show

184

the hospital as in continuing crisis — an enormous stimulus to fund raising![27]

The need to balance the books led to changes in the rules of the hospital as hard-pressed treasurers looked for ways of reducing expenditure. 'Hotel' costs — the provision of a bed, linen and food to patients — were never less than 53 per cent of total expenditure annually. In 1858 such costs came to over £1,345, 56 per cent, and the rules clearly stated:

> The friends of patients, not exceeding two on the same day to each patient, shall be permitted to visit them on Tuesdays and Fridays, between Two and Four o'Clock, p.m. *They shall bring no provisions (tea and sugar excepted), and shall take none away*; and if detected in so doing, they shall never again be admitted into the Infirmary. After leaving the house, they shall not be allowed to return during the same day[28] (emphasis added).

By the final decades of the nineteenth century, patients were being allowed and often actively encouraged to bring in 'bacon, butter, bread, cake, apples, slices of meat, etc.', as well as bed linen in a few exceptional cases.[29]

THE NEW NURSES AND THEIR COST TO THE HOSPITALS

It was into this context that the new hospital nurses came, at first regarded as unnecessary additional calls on already tight budgets but quickly seen as potential assets in the drive to keep the hospital going financially.[30]

The number of hospital nurses rose from approximately 1,000 in 1861 to over 56,000 in 1921.[31] Brian Abel-Smith is undoubtedly correct in asserting that the major obstacle to the generalised introduction of the new nurses, particularly whilst they were in training, was the cost of the provision of board and lodgings.[32] Those costs were considerable, particularly where the nursing staff was large. Hospital administrators, less than convinced of the need for a different type of nurse, had to face the real problem of housing and feeding them. One way was to use special donations to purchase or adapt existing property and then to name the nurses' home after the donor. This approach to the problem kept the actual costs of providing a building out of the general accounts of the hospital and added to the 'image' of the hospital. Alternatively, totally unsuitable accommodation which might have been left to the hospital in a bequest could be used as a nurses' home.

Costs could be reduced in other ways, such as reducing running costs to an absolute minimum. Whilst some of the more prestigious hospitals — for example, St Thomas's — offered nurses single rooms, many more offered only shared accommodation for at least part of the training period. The nurses were often expected to contribute to the upkeep of the home by carrying out some of the cleaning. Even where they did not actually clean, the discipline under which they lived ensured that they were constantly aware of the need for a 'tidy environment'. In that, they were encouraged by the home sister, who acted as a sort of 'moral police officer'[33]

The daily work of the nurse included many cost-saving tasks. For example, most nurses washed and rolled bandages; most had cleaning duties to perform each day on the wards; many repaired linen or cleaned out cupboards; and many nurses prepared part of the patients' meals in the ward kitchens. Whilst the rhetoric of reformed nursing emphasised the training aspects of such tasks — learning the 'art and science of nursing' as well as self-discipline and early management practices — these were also important ways in which the total costs of running the hospital might be kept down.

In some hospitals, nurses made a more direct and acknowledged contribution to the economic viability of the institution. At the Royal South Hants, for example, the matron contributed to income generation and helped reduce overall expenditure. In addition to her nursing duties, she was also responsible for the kitchens and the domestic staff. The annual reports record that

Table 11.1: Income derived from the work of the matron, RSH

	Matron's wages	Sale of refuse	Donations given directly to nurses
1855	£41 5s 0d	£40 19s 0d	£7 11s 8d
1857	£45 0s 0d	£47 0s 6d	£9 7s 4d
1858	£45 0s 0d	£50 2s 10d	£11 8s 6d
1859	Not available		
1860	£45 0s 0d	£51 12s 10d	£11 9s 2d
1861	£48 15s 0d	£59 4s 10d	£10 18s 2d

she was responsible for selling the kitchen waste or 'refuse'. Just how important she was to the hospital is shown in the table.

But like the middle class wife, on whom they were modelled, most of the contributions made by the matron and her nurses were hidden from public view. One such contribution was the use of time. The old nurses — the gamps — were castigated for their *waste* of time; the new nurses were characterised by their *use* of time.[34] And it was not just that the new discipline regime made nurses stay on duty until their allotted tasks were completed. The introduction of shift work, an event hardly noticed by historians of nursing, helped to get the last crumb of effort out of the new nurses.[35]

In time, hospital administrators recognised the value of having the new nurses on the wards but at about the same moment they also realised the potential income which could accrue if they sold the labour of the nurses outside the institution. The growth of private duty staffs in most voluntary hospitals has been discussed elsewhere;[36] as contemporaries like Sir Henry Burdett — himself one of the earliest of the new generation of professional hospital administrators — were quick to realise, the demand for private nurses for the middle classes was apparently, insatiable. Burdett claimed that London Hospital was getting nearly £4,000 net from its private nursing staff: in his view, the hospitals were taking from the new generation of nurses 'with both hands'.[37]

CONCLUSION

We have argued that the existence of the hospital was a fragile affair and that considerable effort was constantly expended on maintaining its economic survival. It has been suggested that many of the characteristics which were said to set the new nurses apart from the old, prereform nurses are capable of interpretation as part of that process. That is not to say that this was the sole reason for the introduction and acceptance of the new nurses. However, there are no neutral 'facts' in the development of nursing and to see the evolution of nursing separate from other changes leads to error. We have not examined the many other ways in which the hospital and the new nurses interacted with the local economies. For example, the importance of new employment opportunities for single women in the urban areas has to be recognised.

187

In a single year, 1891, the voluntary hospitals together spent £326,000 on provisions; £129,000 on surgery and dispensary items; £172,000 on cleaning and laundries; and £268,000 on wages.[38] Much, if not all, of that entered local economies. Hamilton has, therefore, a point: hospitals are and were crucial to the local and national economies apart from their roles as medical institutions, and his analysis of the 1960s finds an earlier echo in our period. And the Hollingsworths are undoubtedly correct in their analysis of the collapse of the voluntary hospital system in the interwar period which opened the way for the National Health Service. This paper has suggested that the seeds of that collapse were sown in the mid-nineteenth century and that nursing was part of that process.

NOTES

An earlier version of this paper was given to a conference on new perspectives in nursing history, King's Fund Centre, London, July 1983 and to the Staff Seminar, Department of Humanities, Bristol Polytechnic, England in May 1984. I am grateful for the comments and suggestions made by participants on both occasions.

1. J. A. Hamilton et al., Patterns of hospital ownership and control (Oxford University Press, London, 1961), p.9.

2. R. and E. J. Hollingsworth, 'Voluntary and public hospitals in England and Wales', unpublished paper, University of Wisconsin, 1983.

3. B. Abel-Smith, The hospitals 1800–1948: a study in social administration in England and Wales (Heinemann, London, 1964); see also, R. Pinker, English hospital statistics 1861–1938 (Heinemann, London, 1966).

4. The seminal work in this area is M. Foucault, The birth of the clinic: an archeology of medical perception (Tavistock, London, 1976).

5. D. M. Watson, Proud heritage: a history of the Royal South Hants Hospital, 1838–1971 (Wilson, Southampton, 1979).

6. Ruth Hawker, 'For the good of the patient', supra, Chapter Nine.

7. F. N. L. Poynter (ed.), The evolution of hospitals in Britain (Pitman, London, 1964), p.43.

8. J. E. Stone, Hospital organisation and management (Faber, London, 1952), p.4.

9. Poynter (ed.), The evolution of hospitals in Britain, p.48.

10. J. Woodward, 'To do the Sick no harm': a study of the British voluntary hospital system to 1875 (Routledge and Kegan Paul, London, 1974) (1978 edn), p.18; Abel-Smith, The hospitals 1800–1948, p.5.

11. Abel-Smith, The hospitals 1800–1948, p.1.

12. However, see the Annual Reports of the Royal South Hants Infirmary, 1855–1861 where length of stay and crude bed-occupancy rates are given. Archives of the Royal South Hants Infirmary, The Hospital,

Southampton.

13. Pinker, *English hospital statistics*, pp.48–49; p.57; p.61; Abel-Smith, *The hospitals 1800–1948*, p.102.

14. Abel-Smith, *The hospitals 1800–1948*, pp.21–31.

15. Data in this section are taken from the *Annual Reports of the Royal South Hants Infirmary*, 1855–61.

16. 'Abstract of the rules', *Annual Report of the Royal South Hants Infirmary for 1858*, p.9.

17. Ibid.

18. Watson, *Proud heritage*.

19. *Annual Report of the Royal South Hants Infirmary for 1859*, pp.7–8.

20. *Annual Report of the Royal South Hants Infirmary for 1860*, p.5.

21. Ibid., p.6; p.23.

22. Stone, *Hospital organisation and management* , p.6.

23. Abel-Smith, *The hospitals 1800–1948*, p.33.

24. Pinker, *English hospital statistics*, p.143.

25. Ibid.

26. Ibid.

27. Ibid.

28. 'Abstract of the rules', *Annual Report of the Royal South Hants Infirmary for 1858*, p.10.

29. Abel-Smith, *The hospitals 1800–1948*, p.43; Pinker, *English hospital statistics*, p.150.

30. C. J. Maggs, *Origins of general nursing* (Croom Helm, London, 1983), Chapter 4; C. J. Maggs, 'Control mechanisms and the "new nurses", 1881–1914', *Nursing Times* (2 September 1981).

31. Maggs, *Origins of general nursing*, pp.6–9.

32. Abel-Smith, *The hospitals 1800–1948*, p.67.

33. Maggs, *Origins of general nursing*, p.112.

34. Maggs, *Origins of general nursing*, pp.107–12; pp.122–6; p.193.

35. Ibid., Chapter 3.

36. Ibid., pp.85–5; pp. 153–5.

37. Abel-Smith, *A history of the nursing profession* (Heinemann, London, 1960), p.51.

38. Stone, *Hospital organisation and management*. In 1891 the total income of the voluntary hospitals exceeded £17,800,000; in 1911 it was more than £31,000,000. The figures for expenditure in 1911 are: £435,000 on provisions; £226,000 for surgery and dispensary items; £327,000 on cleaning and laundries; and £509,000 for wages.

Index